The Other Diabetes

The Other Diabetes

LIVING AND EATING WELL
WITH TYPE 2 DIABETES

♥

Elizabeth Hiser

WM

WILLIAM MORROW
An Imprint of HarperCollins*Publishers*

HarperCollins books may be purchased for educational, business, or sales promotional use. For information, please write to: Special Markets Department, HarperCollins Publishers Inc., 10 East 53rd Street, New York, NY 10022.

Grateful acknowledgment is made for permission to reprint "The Traditional Healthy Mediterranean Diet Pyramid," copyright © 1994 by Oldways Preservation & Trust.

Book design by Gretchen Achilles.

First William Morrow paperback edition published 2002.

Library of Congress cataloging-in-publication data

Hiser, Elizabeth.
The other diabetes : living and eating well with type 2 diabetes / Elizabeth Hiser.—1st pbk. ed.
p. cm.
Includes bibliographical references and index.
ISBN 0-06-008813-3
1. Non-insulin-dependent diabetes—Popular works. I. Title.
RC662.18.H56 2002
616.4'62—dc21
2001056219

03 04 05 QW 10 9 8 7 6 5 4 3 2

This book is dedicated to my grandmother,

EUPHAMIA CAMPBELL RENDALL,

and to my first mentor,

DR. ETHAN ALLEN SIMS

♥

Contents

♥

About This Book

Today, help with type 2 diabetes depends largely on the luck of the draw. If you live near a diabetes clinic with a great staff and a support group of people who are working on the same problem, you are indeed fortunate. If not, you are on your own, and this means you could be getting lots of advice from well-meaning friends and relatives who think you will be okay if you stay away from sugar. What you need is a plan and, ideally, the help of health professionals to support you along the way. But keep in mind that people who do the best at lifestyle changes, such as losing weight or quitting smoking, are those who use the resources available and take responsibility for their own health.

This book is one such resource. It is your guide to understanding how diet and exercise work to control type 2 diabetes, and it is your guide for creating your own plan. And because understanding the problem is the first step to dealing with it, several chapters are devoted to explaining how things work in the body and what goes wrong in type 2 diabetes. But if you find the information too detailed—or if you already have a good understanding of how things work—it is fine to cut to the chase and start using the diet and exercise plans. The information is there when you need it. For example, if you want to know exactly why eating high-fiber bread is good for your weight, blood sugar, and cholesterol, you can go back and read about the research that backs this up. Or if you want to be inspired to do a little weight lifting, you can learn why investing just a few minutes a day can give you a great payback.

I have devoted the largest part of the book to nutrition because what to eat and why is such a rich and varied topic, and I have made my career out of helping people bring nutrition to the table. The good news is that you will not be on a "diabetic diet"; your healthy way of eating can be shared by family and friends to lower *their* risk of type 2 diabetes, heart disease, obesity, and cancer. The recipes and meal plans are examples of how to translate the science of eating well to actual food choices.

I am a registered dietitian and a writer with a long-standing interest in type 2 diabetes. My goal is to show you what is important, what isn't important, and how to put it all together in a plan you can live with. To help *me* put it all together, I asked my good friend and fellow dietitian, Robin Edelman, who is a certified diabetes educator, to review and add her thoughts to the book. I have also called upon other experts—researchers, clinicians, educators, and the most important experts of all, people like you who have battled the disease and won.

—E.H.

♥

CHAPTER 1

The Other Diabetes

Although people usually think diabetes is caused by a lack of insulin, the hormone that lowers blood sugar, more often than not the disease is characterized by too much rather than too little insulin. In fact, nine out of ten cases in the United States are type 2 (adult-onset) diabetes, which typically starts out with high insulin levels. But people are usually more familiar with the less-common type 1 (insulin-requiring) diabetes, because it is an immediate threat to life: If you don't get insulin you die. The *other* diabetes is more insidious—half of the people who have type 2 diabetes don't even know it. As expert Dr. James Gavin puts it, type 2 diabetes "takes its victims a little piece at a time."

Too much body fat sets the stage for type 2 diabetes by decreasing the body's ability to use insulin. As we all well know, extra fat is the result of taking in more calories than we burn, which means that too much food and too little exercise are big contributors to type 2 diabetes. But not everyone with a spare tire gets type 2 diabetes; genetics also plays a role. And from the current epidemic—an estimated sixteen million cases nationwide—it appears that the underlying genetic tendency is not all that rare.

To understand why type 2 diabetes is becoming more common, it helps to step back and take a look at the big picture—where and when the disease occurs. If you have type 2 diabetes, you are not alone. By the year

2000, experts predict that the epidemic we are seeing in the United States will have spread worldwide. How could this be when we are talking about an inherited disorder, not a contagious disease? What *is* contagious is technology, which creates the environment that causes the disease to surface.

Type 2 diabetes is widespread in industrialized nations, such as the United States, the United Kingdom, and Finland, whereas nations with third world economies, as in parts of Asia and Africa, do not have such epidemics. "If you look at the spread of the scourge around the world, type 2 diabetes occurs as a country advances technologically, when people come out of the fields and sit behind desks," say Dr. Irwin Brodsky. Brodsky, a diabetes researcher and clinician who directs the Diabetes Treatment Center at the University of Illinois at Chicago, explains, "It's almost a sign of coming of age; in Saudi Arabia, for example, where oil money started flowing in the late sixties and seventies, we saw a blip in the occurrence of type 2 diabetes about ten years later." Simply said, too much food and too little activity are pushing more and more people with the underlying tendency for type 2 diabetes over the edge.

An industrial economy is a double-edged sword, providing a calorie-rich food supply with little need for physical work to bring home the bacon. Technological advances such as refrigeration, improved agricultural techniques, better transportation, and food processing plants all help make more food readily available to most of the world's population. Initially, these advances have a positive impact on a nation's health by feeding the hungry; but eventually, a richer food supply leads to new health problems.

A CENTURY OF PROGRESS

Before the Industrial Revolution, food was often scarce, and what was available did not always provide the balance of nutrients needed to prevent deficiency diseases. In nineteenth-century England, for example, hundreds of thousands of children died of malnutrition. Among the poor, bread, potatoes, and porridge provided the bulk of the calories. Often the only meat was a small bit of bacon cut up with the potatoes; the poorest subsisted on potatoes alone. Those who survived on the poverty-line diet often suffered from scurvy, a deficiency of vitamin C from the lack of fresh fruits and vegetables; rickets, from lack of sunlight and vitamin D; and tuberculosis, a bacterial infection that thrives in a malnourished host. When the great potato famine hit in the 1840s, poor Irish and English immigrants came to America, where there was plenty of land and a promising new agricultural economy.

As homesteaders were given the opportunity to grow their own food on their own land, wave upon wave of immigrants settled farther and farther west. It was a hard life, and the diet of the settlers was one of subsistence based on easily transportable foods that would keep. The typical meal in Laura Ingalls Wilder's memoir *Little House on the Prairie* consisted of coffee, cornmeal cakes, and salt pork. She described a special meal that her family shared around 1880:

> There was stewed jack rabbit with white-flour dumplings and plenty of gravy. There was a steaming-hot, thick cornbread flavored with bacon fat. There was molasses to eat on the cornbread, but because this was company supper, they did not sweeten their coffee with molasses. Ma brought out the little paper sack of pale-brown store sugar.

Don't be fooled by the bit of bacon fat and sugar; the extra calories provided by such meals were still barely enough to sustain a hardworking frontier family. Today, a special meal is likely to include several courses; generous servings of meat, drinks, and dessert; and needless to say, many times more calories than meals served in an era when work was physical and type 2 diabetes was unknown.

After the Civil War and the Industrial Revolution, the need to provide more food for the expanding population spawned a wave of technological advances. By the 1890s, there were improved canning, flour milling, plant breeding, and refrigeration techniques as well as new disease-resistant varieties of wheat and the first gasoline-driven tractors. In the 1920s, Clarence Birdseye introduced a method for freezing produce; by the 1960s, we had high-powered machinery, new fertilizers and pesticides, poultry raised in completely controlled environments, new breeds of heat-resistant cattle, McDonald's burgers and fries, and the heart disease epidemic. In 1983, one in four Americans was overweight; in 1995, it became one in three. From 1958 to 1993, the incidence of type 2 diabetes tripled. All in all, it had taken about a hundred years for overnutrition to become as big a killer as undernutrition.

A MATTER OF NATURE *and* NURTURE

We have to go back even further in time and look at the *really* big picture to understand why the underlying tendency for type 2 diabetes is so common. The bodies we have today work the same way as did those of our prehistoric ancestors. Only our environment—including what we eat and how we live—is different. But the bodily systems that keep us alive by managing energy and nutrients evolved through natural selection during a time when survival of the fit meant being able to stay alive on as little food as possible.

From about 3.5 million years ago to 8000 B.C., we were completely at the mercy of nature. As members of wandering groups, we had to stay on the move to find food, because we had not yet developed the knowledge to plant seeds and wait for the harvest. We hunted, fished, and gathered food to stay alive. Even after we learned to plant crops and domesticate animals, great famines wiped out entire populations. But it was during the period of hunting and gathering that our finely tuned physiology evolved, allowing our ancestors to survive periods of starvation. And key to their survival was the ability to store energy in the form of body fat.

Fat is dense, compact, and transportable, exactly the type of stored fuel needed to stay on the move in search of the next meal. In fact, the pre-humans who were most efficient in storing body fat had the distinct advantage over other those who were less efficient—the skinny guys—because they could live for longer periods of time without eating. So according to Darwin's theory of natural selection, many of our ancestors became pretty good in the fat-storing department or they wouldn't have lived to reproduce. (Females became even better than males because they had to store enough energy for two.)

All in all, it is not surprising that people can easily gain too much weight when there is extra food around just waiting to be eaten—our brains are hard-wired to go after calories, and our bodies are geared to store them up in case of famine. Unfortunately, what was a good thing throughout most of human history is now a problem for many people. And just as weight gain is more of a problem for some people than for others, type 2 diabetes is more of a problem for some people, most of whom have also had to battle their weight. Researchers suspect that the genes that cause people to store fat very efficiently may also predispose them to type 2 diabetes.

AN UNWELCOME INHERITANCE

You may already be aware that Americans of African, Mexican, Hawaiian, and Native American descent are more likely to experience type 2 diabetes and obesity than the population as a whole; and this appears to be connected to inherited tendencies. Worldwide, there are other pockets of people with common gene pools in which type 2 diabetes runs rampant, whereas more heterogeneous population groups get the disease less frequently. Since the 1960s, researchers have been studying the Pima Indians of Arizona, a group of Native Americans with the highest rate of type 2 diabetes in the world.

Once a lean and vigorous people, the Pima Indians are believed to have descended from the Hohokam, a group of Paleo-Indians who originally came from Asia during the first of the great migrations across the Bering land bridge. The Hohokam first settled in what is now northern Mexico; and around 300 B.C., a group migrated to the Gila River valley in what is now Arizona. For more than two thousand years, the ancestors of the present-day Pimas lived in the desert environment by irrigation farming, hunting, and gathering food. They built elaborate irrigation systems, diverting water to cultivated fields, and lived successfully until the end of the nineteenth century when their water supplies were disrupted by white settlers.

In this century, health changes have followed cultural and economic changes. Compared to children at the turn of the century, present-day Pima children are much heavier for their height. Today, one out of two Pimas under the age of thirty-five has type 2 diabetes, and about 90 percent of the adults are obese.

Researchers study the Pimas to understand the interrelationships among obesity and type 2 diabetes, genetics, and environment. With an adult obesity rate of about 90 percent, it is clear that the Pimas have been influenced by access to a calorically dense diet and the fact that hard physical labor is no longer a way of life. But because this can be said about almost the entire North American population, why are some groups more severely affected than others? It may be that the Pimas' long history of survival through famines and a harsh environment had been possible because of a genetic tendency to store fat efficiently.

The existence of the so-called thrifty gene was predicted nearly thirty years ago, and the puzzle of the Pima legacy has been carefully studied. Indeed, differences in metabolism and fat storage that contribute to obesity have been documented at a Phoenix-based diabetes research station funded by the National Institutes of Health.

But in spite of the powerful effect of genes, it appears that lifestyle is the determining factor for who will and will not get type 2 diabetes. When Phoenix researchers went to the highlands of northern Mexico to study indigenous peoples who share a common ancestry with the Pimas, they found striking differences. Adult male Pimas, who live on reservations with high rates of unemployment, have an average weight of about 200 pounds and suffer terribly from the ravages of type 2 diabetes. The disease is virtually unknown among their Mexican counterparts, who live in the rugged mountains, gathering and growing their own food, and who weigh an average of about 130 pounds.

GENE SEARCH

Dr. Bo Bogardus, a National Institutes of Health researcher who has worked with the Pimas for nearly fifteen years, is committed to helping solve their plight with type 2 diabetes. "Genetics is going to be the answer," says Bogardus, "but resolving this is not going to be quick and easy."

The search is complicated because, unlike diseases such as cystic fibrosis and Huntington disease for which just one gene is the culprit, even the most common forms of type 2 diabetes may be caused by three, four, or even five genes. The group of mutant genes interact with each other and the environment, leading to the expression of type 2 diabetes.

One clue has been the discovery of the "obesity gene," which produces leptin. When this fat-burning hormone was cloned and injected into genetically obese mice, the animals became thin. The so-called OB mouse has a look-alike cousin, the DB mouse, who is not only obese but also develops type 2 diabetes. However, because the DB mouse has plenty of leptin (and so do the Pimas tested so far), the problem appears to be leptin resistance. Because leptin is an important protein that tells the brain when you've stored enough fat and it's time to stop eating, could leptin resistance go hand in hand with insulin resistance? "This question remains to be answered," says Bogardus. "But we're sure working on it."

THE ROOT OF THE PROBLEM: INSULIN RESISTANCE

Although researchers may still have a way to go to completely understand the genetics of type 2 diabetes, they do know that insulin resistance is the hallmark of the disease. Insulin resistance occurs when too much body fat impairs the body's ability to use insulin. Lowering body fat lowers insulin resistance.

Insulin is a hormone secreted by the beta cells in the pancreas in response to eating. As food travels from the mouth to the stomach, enzymes along the way break down the carbohydrates into glucose, which is absorbed into the bloodstream from the small intestine. The rising levels of blood glucose signal the beta cells to secrete insulin. The main job of insulin is to move blood sugar (glucose) into cells where it can be used as energy. Every second of every day, cells need energy to stay alive; and glucose, the basic product of carbohydrate digestion, is a primary source of energy.

Cells are encased in a protective covering, a semipermeable membrane that regulates the entry and exit of substances into and out of the cell. Normally, insulin docks with insulin receptors on the cell membrane, which is the signal to allow glucose to pass through. But in a state of insulin resistance, the receptors do not respond properly to insulin, which causes glucose to back up in the blood. When blood glucose stays a little higher than normal between meals and in the fasting state, a person is said to have impaired glucose tolerance. Impaired glucose tolerance is common in older individuals, particularly those who are sedentary, and in younger people who are overweight. When blood sugar stays a lot higher than normal between meals and in the fasting state, a diagnosis of type 2 diabetes is made.

In type 2 diabetes, blood sugar stays high between meals even though insulin levels remain high, which is a sure sign that cells are responding poorly to insulin's signal. A person in this situation is said to be in a state of insulin resistance. The goal for managing type 2 diabetes is to increase insulin sensitivity, so that insulin's signal is readily received, allowing glucose to be effectively cleared from the blood.

SENSITIVITY RAISING

Why do cells lose their insulin sensitivity? It was once believed that too much fat stored in fat cells caused distortions in the insulin receptors, but this does not explain why muscle and liver cells also lose their sensitivity. Scientists have yet to unravel the exact biochemical chain of events that cells use to regulate the entry of glucose. But by studying people with and without type 2 diabetes, they do know that there are several ways to increase insulin sensitivity:

- **Stem the flood of calories.** Too much insulin and glucose can be looked on as the result of taking in more food than the body can effectively manage, so cutting back lessens the burden. In fact, at one time, doctors put people on complete fasts or modified fasts as a way of bringing down blood sugar levels that were wildly out of control. But we now know that fasting can be dangerous and more moderate cutbacks are much more likely to lead to long-term success.

- **Start moving.** Any type of activity, even combing your hair or washing the dishes, helps with insulin sensitivity. This is because muscle cells, the body's biggest energy users, need the assistance of insulin to get more fuel. Exercise really has a double benefit: It makes cells pay better attention to insulin and it burns body fat, which helps raise insulin sensitivity both in the short run and in the long run.

- **Eat a reasonable amount of carbohydrates.** It may seem ironic that carbohydrates, which are often blamed for causing diabetes, are actually necessary for maximizing insulin sensitivity. This is why people are told to "carbohydrate load" before a glucose-tolerance test. Of course, this does not mean that loading up on excess calories from carbohydrates is a good idea; it means that the ideal diet contains the right amount of calories from a balance of carbohydrates, fats, and protein. Insulin resistance comes from too high a calorie burden and not necessarily from too many carbohydrates.

Although most cells of the body have insulin receptors as gatekeepers, certain cells, such as those of the blood, kidneys, and central nervous system, do not need insulin to take in glucose. This may be a protective feature that allows the critical cells of the brain, for example, to get enough glucose whether or not insulin is present and whether or not it is working properly. But a different problem occurs when blood glucose stays high: Over time, these insulin-independent cells can be damaged by the constant spillover of excess glucose. Overcoming insulin resistance and keeping blood glucose in control protects the eyes, kidneys, and nerve cells from the effects of too much glucose.

Weight loss lowers insulin resistance. And although it is obvious that diet and exercise are the ways to lose weight, you should know that the composition of the diet and the type of exercise have other beneficial effects on insulin resistance. This book will tell you all about the composition of the ideal diet for type 2 diabetes, a diet that includes fats known to have beneficial health effects in moderate amounts. The type of fat you eat is so important that we will refer to this healthy and satisfying approach to eating as the Good Fat Diet. This book will also show you how to make exercise work for you. But first let's look at the most pressing reason for overcoming insulin resistance now: heart disease.

CHAPTER 2

Public Enemy Number One:
Heart Disease

You probably already know that heart disease kills more Americans than does any other disease, but you may not know that uncontrolled type 2 diabetes multiplies heart disease risk by as much as five times. Both men *and women* with type 2 diabetes develop heart disease at a younger age than the rest of the population; and when a heart attack strikes, they are twice as likely to die within six months as people without diabetes. The hard cold fact is that our nation's number one killer is also the number one reason for preventing or taking control of type 2 diabetes now.

Yet even the experts have only recently become aware of how much type 2 diabetes magnifies the risk of heart disease. In fact, recognizing the seriousness of the problem is one of the moving forces behind recent public health campaigns to educate everyone about type 2 diabetes. The goal is to get more people diagnosed earlier, because damage to arteries usually begins long before most people even know they have the disease.

WHAT YOU SHOULD KNOW ABOUT HEART DISEASE

The best way to fight heart disease is to first understand what goes on in the body and what can go wrong. First of all, genes—including some of the same genes that make people prone to type 2 diabetes—have a strong influence on heart disease risk. Although scientists have barely begun to understand the many inherited glitches that contribute to heart disease—*why* things go wrong—they do have a good idea of *what* goes wrong. There is no doubt that a direct cause is the accumulation of fatty deposits, or **plaque,** on the inner walls of arteries. The buildup of plaque is called **atherosclerosis,** from the Greek word *athero* for "gruel" or "paste," and *sclerosis,* meaning "hardness." Plaque interferes with blood flow through arteries, which can become blocked when a blood clot forms on the plaque's surface. A blood clot that breaks off and/or a complete blockage can cause a heart attack or stroke. (For the purposes of this book, the term *heart disease* is used for "cardio-vascular disease," which includes risk of both heart attack and stroke.)

If you're wondering if it is important to understand how arteries become damaged, consider this: Atherosclerosis accounts for about 80 percent of deaths from diabetes.

Atherosclerosis is a slow process that is believed to start during child-hood and progress throughout life. Artery damage moves ahead more rapidly in some people than in others, and researchers have spent decades trying to find out why. What they have concentrated on most is learning about the carriers in the body that transport fats and cholesterol in the blood and how they affect the arteries through which they travel. These protein carriers are called **lipoproteins** (fat proteins).

BEYOND CHOLESTEROL: OTHER NEW CLUES TO HEART DISEASE

Although keeping lipoproteins and triglycerides at healthy levels is still the top priority for fighting heart disease, researchers have now discovered that arteries can be damaged in other ways as well.

Homocysteine. Homocysteine, a substance in the blood that is neither fat nor cholesterol, has also been linked to heart disease. But don't be dis-couraged by yet another scientific-sounding name and something else to worry about; this time the news is good, because there may be an easy solution to the problem. Homocysteine is a small bit of protein, actually an amino acid, or protein building block. After a meal, protein is broken down to its amino acids, including methionine, which is converted to homocysteine. Normally, homocysteine levels stay low because it is regularly used to make other amino acids. But sometimes homocysteine levels become high, and nearly thirty years ago, a medical researcher named Kilmer McCully discovered that high homocysteine levels damage artery walls. Unfortunately, he was laughed at by the medical establishment, which believed that blood cholesterol was the only problem. Well, they're not laughing now: Several large health studies have supported McCully's research, and some experts say that high homocysteine levels should be classified as a risk factor for heart disease, just like smoking or high cholesterol. The encouraging news is that, in most people, keeping homocysteine levels where they should be may be as easy as getting enough vitamins (Chapter 9).

Infections. New research suggests that bloodborne infections, such as those that begin with periodontal (gum) disease and certain types of respiratory illnesses, may inflame and damage arteries. It appears that bacteria can set up housekeeping along artery walls, which can lead to plaque formation from deposits of bacteria and cells sent from the immune system to fight them. Other new research suggests that aspirin protects against heart disease because it is an anti-inflammatory agent. (It was previously believed that aspirin's protection came solely from its ability to prevent blood clots.) These new findings suggest that it is important to take care of your teeth and gums, to keep your immune system strong with good nutrition, and to talk to your doctor about aspirin therapy.

Low birth weight. A growing body of evidence suggests that poor maternal nutrition during pregnancy has a profound influence on the child's health as an adult. Babies whose birth weight is less than 5.5 pounds have a 35 percent higher rate of coronary death later in life. Low birth weight also predisposes an individual to type 2 diabetes.

LIPOPROTEINS: THE GOOD, THE BAD, AND THE UGLY

From meal to meal, calories that are not used are stored as fat. The liver assembles the leftovers into fat particles to ready them for shipping and storage. Because fat does not mix with water, the fat particles get a coating of water-soluble protein before they enter the bloodstream. These tiny transport vehicles, called lipoproteins, carry cholesterol as well, and they take different forms in the blood.

One type of lipoprotein is **high-density lipoprotein** (HDL), also known as the "good cholesterol," because it picks up cholesterol and carries it away from artery walls. High HDL levels are strongly linked with protection against heart disease. In general, women tend to have higher HDL levels than do men, because estrogen raises them. This is one way estrogen protects premenopausal women and postmenopausal women who take hormone-replacement therapy against heart disease.

MAXIMIZE THE POSITIVE

Your HDL level is largely determined by genetics, but there are ways to keep it as high as possible through

1. Exercise.

2. Monounsaturated fats.

3. Moderate alcohol consumption.

4. Prescription drugs and hormone-replacement therapy.

The other main type of lipoprotein is **low-density lipoprotein** (LDL). Also known as the "bad cholesterol," LDLs are the kind that end up in artery-clogging plaque. How well the body handles lipoprotein traffic is in part determined by genetics; but LDL levels are also strongly influenced by diet, particularly by the type of fat eaten. Eating saturated fats causes LDLs to rise; replacing saturated fats with monounsaturated and polyunsaturated fats causes LDLs to fall.

But in recent years, researchers have reached a new understanding of how LDLs damage artery walls and cause plaque formation. They now believe that LDLs become far more dangerous when they are oxidized. Oxidation is a process that is fundamental to life; but it also produces harmful by-products called **free radicals**, which travel in the bloodstream looking for something to oxidize. Because fat is easily oxidized, fat-laden LDLs are the perfect target. In turn, oxidized LDLs become toxic to the cells lining artery walls; and when they come in contact with them, the immune system sends special scavenger cells to gobble up the oxidized LDLs and take them away. But the immune system can't always keep up. When there are too many oxidized LDLs to handle, a vicious circle ensues: Scavenger cells stuffed full of bad cholesterol take up residence in the artery wall; next, sensing that the artery has been damaged, surrounding muscle cells begin to multiply. Soon sticky cells designed for blood clotting become snagged in the debris, and wave after wave of immune cells are sent to the rescue.

Here's an easy way to remember which lipoprotein is which: Think H for healthy or HDL, the good cholesterol; think for lousy or LDL, the b cholesterol.

Because oxidation is the cause of these nasty pileups, antioxidants—defenses that keep oxidation in check—should help prevent them. Research suggests they do. Vitamin E, the now-famous antioxidant vitamin, hitches a ride on LDL particles, where it protects against oxidation. Dozens of studies have suggested that this is how vitamin E protects arteries (page 72). And although we're still waiting for the results of long-term trials, most experts are now so confident that research will confirm vitamin E as a weapon against heart disease that they themselves take vitamin E. There is also new evidence that vitamin C, another antioxidant vitamin, assists vitamin E in protecting LDLs by patrolling the bloodstream and disarming free radicals before they can attack.

In people with diabetes, the arteries are also damaged by high blood sugar because of glucose's tendency to link up with proteins to form **glycated proteins.** Surplus glucose molecules can hook up with the protein part of lipoproteins, and glycated LDLs are more easily snagged along artery walls. Proteins in cells lining artery walls are also vulnerable to this type of glucose damage.

Triglyceride is another name for the fat that is carried on lipoproteins, and triglycerides tend to rise with weight gain. It is not known if triglycerides damage arteries directly; but there is new evidence that they are another risk factor for heart disease, particularly when accompanied by low HDL levels, as they often are in people with type 2 diabetes. In fact, there is a syndrome, or group of symptoms, typically found in people with type 2 diabetes and underlying heart disease. And because heart disease kills far more people with type 2 diabetes than all of the other complications combined, it is important to know about this cluster of symptoms, which is called syndrome X or insulin resistance syndrome.

INSULIN RESISTANCE SYNDROME

Most people with type 2 diabetes and heart disease are different from people with heart disease alone: Instead of high LDLs, they tend to have more moderately elevated LDLs, accompanied by low HDLs and high triglycerides. They often have a group of related problems that reseachers believe are all linked to insulin resistance. Insulin resistance syndrome greatly raises heart disease risk.

High blood pressure. Hypertension is common in people diagnosed with type 2 diabetes, and researchers suspect it is connected to insulin resistance. Hypertension increases the risk of heart attack or stroke because it puts more strain on the heart and blood vessels.

Central distribution of body fat. Extra weight that's carried above the waist rather than in the hips and thighs is associated with a risk of both type 2 diabetes and heart disease.

Low HDL levels. The way fat is carried on the inside affects heart disease risk for everyone, and unfortunately low HDLs are one of the hallmarks of insulin resistance syndrome.

High triglycerides. Elevated triglycerides are now believed to raise everyone's risk of heart disease, and they are definitely more dangerous when combined with low HDLs.

Small dense LDLs. Although high LDL levels are not necessarily a sign of insulin resistance syndrome, there may be an association with small dense LDLs, a type of LDL that is more easily oxidized than are normal LDLs.

A SILENT KILLER

The fact that undiagnosed type 2 diabetes is so widespread has led researchers to begin referring to the problem as a "silent" epidemic or a "silent" killer. And it's the accompanying heart disease that they're most worried about. According to Dr. Richard Nesto, a heart disease prevention specialist at Harvard Medical School, "Too many patients with diabetes are diagnosed with coronary artery disease when it is too far advanced and can no longer be aggressively treated because of years of silent heart damage." A major problem, according to Nesto, is that diabetes patients with nerve damage often do not have chest pain (angina), which normally is a warning to get treatment before a heart attack occurs. Don't wait for chest pain: Ask your doctor to refer you to a heart disease specialist for an evaluation now.

On the positive side, individuals at risk for type 2 diabetes may have more to gain by seeing a specialist than do people who don't have diabetes as a risk factor. The drugs used to treat heart disease, including aspirin, prevent heart attacks and improve survival after a heart attack even more in people with diabetes. Break the silence and get the help you need.

♥

CHAPTER 3

How to Lose Weight and Keep It Off

Now that heart disease has been identified as your number one enemy, it's time to focus on the number one priority for controlling type 2 diabetes. What really matters more than anything else is losing enough weight to lower insulin resistance. Granted, this is not easy; the fact that you may have an inherited tendency for storing calories means that you probably have to push hard to change the status quo. But it is doable, and the rewards are great.

Often losing just ten or twenty pounds is enough, which means that you don't necessarily have to reach some "ideal" weight listed on a weight chart. (Some perfectly healthy people never do.) And once you lose enough to lower your blood sugar and worry less about heart disease, you will truly feel more energized, because your energy will be put to good use.

ENERGY BALANCE

Understanding the energy balance is the first step to understanding how to control type 2 diabetes. The facts are quite simple:

energy stored = energy in − energy out

The word *energy* is interchangeable with the word *calorie,* and it is a good idea to remind yourself that the body is like a furnace that burns energy as fuel. Like heating oil, body fat is a pure, concentrated form of stored energy. Your goal will be to lower the fuel in your storage tank by taking in less and burning more.

As a group, fat, protein, and carbohydrates—the energy nutrients—provide the fuel for the obvious jobs of keeping us warm and giving us power to do our daily activities. But quite a bit of their energy is also used for maintenance jobs, such as keeping the various organ systems running. Each and every cell needs energy to keep it alive, which brings up an important fact of life: Even at rest, muscle cells need more energy to keep them going than do fat cells.

Energy In

To understand the "energy in" part of the equation, take a look at the relative proportions of protein, carbohydrates, and fat in the foods we eat. Food comes from two sources: plants and animals. Plant foods contain all three energy nutrients and most animal foods (except milk and milk products) contain protein and fat, but no carbohydrates. In their natural form, plant foods take up a lot of space for the amount of energy they contain, because they are full of fiber, which does not supply digestible calories. You might say that fiber-containing foods are low in calories per square inch. On the other hand, foods from animal sources are higher in calories per square inch, because they do not contain fiber, yet contain a high proportion of fat, which takes up less space and has more calories than either protein or carbohydrates.

So why is the space issue such a big deal? Well, it gets back to the energy balance and whether you're in an environment where there's too much food or too little food. The stomach can hold only so much; and there's a limit to the amount we can eat, digest, and assimilate into our bodies over any given amount of time. If, for example, you're on an arctic expedition hiking twenty miles a day in subzero temperatures, you want highly concentrated food, namely high-fat foods, because your calorie needs are great and must be met by what you can carry with you. When you are in a cozy comfortable environment and you want to lose weight, the opposite is true: You need to eat foods that are less energy dense and that still make you feel satisfied, namely high-fiber foods.

We are surrounded by fiber-poor, energy-rich foods that taste good. And they taste good to us for a reason. When early humans were foraging for food, it was an evolutionary advantage to develop a taste for concentrated calories: fatty and sweet foods. Indeed, our bodies are still hardwired to go after concentrated calories whenever the opportunity arises. This is why McDonald's restaurants and Coca-Cola are such big hits when they are first introduced in third-world countries.

Energy Out

We also live in a world where we don't have to expend many calories to survive. Even as recently as 150 years ago, when most people had to do hard physical work just to feed themselves, it was an advantage to rest as often as possible. Today, most of us do very little physical work to get food, shelter, and clothing. True, our fingers do get a good workout on the computer and by clicking the television remote control (America *en derrière*), but the other parts of our bodies were designed to move, too. It's those large muscle groups—the ones that transport us from chair to fridge—that need to go farther. The larger the muscle, the more work it is to move it and the more calories it burns.

Every time you move your body, you are fighting against insulin resistance. Your muscles are insulin's biggest target; and the more they're used, the better insulin has to do its job of delivering fuel. And this is exactly the effect you're after.

BALANCING ACT

To help you visualize how to change the energy balance in your favor, take a look at how the body normally goes back and forth between a state of storing calories and a state of burning calories. Insulin and its opposing hormone, glucagon, tell the body what to do with the available energy supply. After a meal, when the blood is carrying more nutrients than the body needs for immediate use, high levels of insulin signal the removal of nutrients from the blood and the storage of fat. Insulin is known as a storage hormone because the body is in a storage state when insulin levels are high.

But fat and glucose (blood sugar) must be made available between meals, because cells need a constant supply of energy. Glucagon tells the body to mobilize some of its fat stores and signals the liver to start making and releasing glucose. (Glucose can be either made from protein or released from glycogen, a storage form of glucose.) Glucagon is the kind of hormone you *want* to have around as often as possible, because it signals the body to draw on its energy stores. When insulin is high, the body is storing fat; when glucagon is high, the body is burning fat.

Here's the rub: When insulin stays high all of the time, as it does with insulin resistance, it is hard for glucagon to get the upper hand and get the fat-burning side rolling. So insulin resistance actually encourages the body to favor the storage mode. What you want to do is get back to a more normal rhythm in which insulin and glucagon are taking turns doing their jobs: storing, burning, storing, burning . . . maybe a little more burning and a little less storing. To make this happen, the body needs to be presented with less food and more physical activity. This is what will lower insulin and insulin resistance.

Your mind is your most powerful tool, so think about these simple priorities for lowering insulin resistance: Eat less, move more. Let this be your mantra.

YOU ARE IN THE DRIVER'S SEAT

In my experience, the mistake people most often make with weight control is depending on some outside force to do it for them. It could be a fad diet, a diet of canned drinks or prepackaged diet foods, or even an exercise gimmick. Given that the weight-control business is a fifteen-billion-dollar industry, there's no end to the possibilities.

But relying on a diet or exercise plan that doesn't really fit into your life means that the weight you lose is bound to come back. It could even happen if you rely too heavily on the meal plans in this book. Say you followed the menus in this book religiously, month after month, even though there were some foods you really didn't like. You would probably lose weight; but because you hadn't adapted the plan to fit your own preferences, you would eventually get tired of it, go back to your old eating habits, and gain all the weight back. The recipes and menus given here are intended to help you get started with your *own* plan.

Another common mistake is thinking that dieting without exercise will keep the weight off. Sure, you can take pounds off with diet alone but you will not be able to keep them off unless you become more active and stay that way. So before we go on to discuss diet, let's explore the meaning of *incorporating more activity into your life,* a phrase you hear all the time. The walking program outlined in the next chapter is certainly a big part of becoming more active. But there are other ways to increase the calories you burn on a daily basis, and it's up to you to decide what works for you. As you have probably guessed by now, in my opinion, the real secret to weight control is being more active all the time, not just once in a while. The bottom line is that it's your body and only you are in the driver's seat. And when you do lose weight, it will be because you made up your mind to do it.

A NEW WORK ETHIC

To begin, let me tell you about the elderly Vermont farmer who used to shake his fist at my husband each time he went by on his daily run. "Waste of good work," he would shout from his perch on the front porch. And he would usually add something like, "Got plenty of hay needs putting up, could use some help." Although his taunts were always good-natured and typical of Vermont humor, he was also making a point. He didn't see the sense of wasting energy that could be put to good use. In his day, body fat—burned by sheer physical labor—was the main energy source for working the farm and running the household. But times have changed; no longer do most people spend a thousand or more calories a day on physical work. Now a person's daily energy expenditure is likely to be a small fraction of that—in many cases not much more than it takes to power fingers across a computer keyboard, a microwave, or Touch-Tone phone.

I would often think of that farmer as I jumped in my car for the thirty-minute drive to my aerobics class. He didn't understand that nowadays we have to make up for time spent sitting at the computer by finding ways to make ourselves exercise. But after my third child was born, it became obvious that my way was no longer working: I simply did not have time to get to my exercise class three times a week, and I was not getting back to my normal weight. With driving and changing time, it was taking me two and a half hours to get one hour of exercise. When I did manage to get to class, my family ate sandwiches for supper and the house was a mess.

When I began to think about ways of fitting in more exercise, I realized that maybe the farmer was right: Wouldn't I be better off doing housework and preparing supper instead of sitting in my car and then jumping around in spandex to make up for all that sitting? So I gave up my health club membership—and saved myself some money, not to mention the stress and worry about trying to get there—and began spending that hour and a half in productive work. I also began walking again, the way I had started out exercising in the first place; but my real breakthrough was finally understanding that any kind of physical work is exercise, and when you do this kind of exercise, you have something to show for it. Now my home is more organized, my family is getting better meals, and I finally lost the weight. I like to think of it as killing two birds with one stone.

But can you really call chopping vegetables and unloading groceries exercise? You bet you can. Compared to sitting on your duff, you burn two to three times as many calories doing household chores, according to careful measurements by exercise experts. In fact, researchers at the Cooper Institute for Aerobics Research in Dallas have even compared the effects of a structured exercise program in the gym to simply adding everyday activities such as walking during work breaks and being more active in general. In their six-month study involving 235 men and women, they found that both the gym group and the home exercise group lowered their blood pressure, improved their blood cholesterol profile, and lost significant amounts of body fat. The improvements were similar between the two groups, but which group do you think found it easier to keep up their exercise after the study ended?

KILL TWO BIRDS WITH ONE STONE: LOSE WEIGHT, GET THINGS DONE

Physical work. Hardly any is required even to meet the most primary of all human needs: getting food into our mouths. But what if it did? According to careful studies of the number of calories burned doing different activities, the average 180-pound person burns 450 calories an hour to get a meal on the table. (It takes him about 180 calories an hour to sit still.) If this doesn't sound like much, how about this? A 180-pound person who currently eats gets all his meals from fast-food places, restaurants, vending machines, and/or by popping a frozen meal in the microwave could lose about twelve pounds in one year if he began preparing food himself, even without consuming fewer calories.

Twelve pounds, just by the physical work it takes to prepare food, assuming that our budding chef spends one hour a day in activities like shopping and cooking. But when the extra calories burned are combined with the potential calories saved by eating home-cooked meals rather than fast food, the weight loss could be even greater. Combine these calorie deficits with thirty minutes of walking each day and now you're really cooking!

Okay, so food preparation may not be the answer for everyone; the point is to spend more time each day being active. First, you need your minimum daily exercise, described in Chapter 4, and then try to engage in other forms of physical work that will help you burn calories and have something to show for it. Think of all the things you've always wanted to do but never got around to, and then pick one that takes some amount of physical effort. It doesn't have to be tap dancing or polo to burn calories; in fact, something less strenuous that you can do at home every day or several times a week will actually fit better into your daily life.

A good example is carpentry. Say you've always wanted to make or refinish furniture, but you've never gotten around to it. Instead, you spend three hours a night in front of the television. Take a Saturday, go out and buy yourself the tools you need, and set up shop in your basement or garage. Now, wouldn't it be a pleasure to spend an hour a night on projects? Never mind the handmade work you would have to show for it—a 180-pound person could lose twelve pounds by doing this five days a week for one year.

Food preparation and carpentry are just two examples. Lawn and garden work is another favorite that can give you great personal satisfaction while helping control your type 2 diabetes. But be creative—playing the drums is a great calorie burner, as is turning pottery. The fact that these activities are not terribly strenuous is not important; as long as they are done on a regular basis, they will help keep weight off. And being involved in something productive will keep you from eating out of boredom.

The important thing is to keep trying until you find activities you enjoy or activities that help get done what needs doing. I always think of my Saturday housecleaning as a way to help me maintain a healthy weight; it's not exactly fun, but it's rewarding because it's good for me and I have a clean house to show for my effort. The chart below will give you an idea of the amount of weight you could lose by adding various activities to your day.

The one rule is that **walking always comes first** because it makes you fitter by making your heart stronger. And this is something you can't do without.

WEIGHT LOSS POTENTIAL FOR ONE YEAR OF ADDED ACTIVITY*

FOOD PREPARATION: 1 hour, 7 days a week
(shopping, putting groceries away, cooking)   12 POUNDS

BRISK WALKING: 30 minutes, 7 days a week
(3.5 miles per hour)   12 POUNDS

CARPENTRY: 1 hour, 5 days a week
(cabinetmaking, sanding, refinishing)   12 POUNDS

YARD WORK: 1 hour, 5 days a week
(mowing, raking, spading, weeding, hoeing)   9 POUNDS

PLAYING THE DRUMS: 1 hour, 3 times a week   10 POUNDS

PLAYING WITH CHILDREN: 30 minutes, 3 times a week
(light activity)   6 POUNDS

FISHING: 1 hour, 2 times a week
(fishing from riverbank, walking)   6 POUNDS

*These numbers are the estimated weight loss for an average 180-pound person, based on 3,500 calories/1 pound of body fat and the energy costs listed in the following source: Ainsworth BE, Haskell WL, Leon AS, et al. Compendium of physical activities: classification of energy costs of human physical activities. *Medicine and Science in Sports and Exercise.* 1995; 25(1):71.

WHERE THERE'S A WILL . . .

I have been lucky enough to hear the stories of hundreds of people who have lost weight and kept it off. A few years ago, I decided I was tired of hearing bad news about weight control—95 percent of dieters gain it all back, yo-yo dieting, binge eating, Americans are getting fatter by the minute—no wonder people were discouraged. I knew there were successes out there, because I had once counseled people who had made up their minds to keep the weight off and did. So when I went to work at *Eating Well* magazine, I decided to use our audience to try to find out more about weight loss success by asking readers who had lost weight and kept it off to write and tell how us they did it.

To my delight, I received nearly 450 letters, and a phone call from a researcher who was looking for answers to the same question. Dr. Jim Hill at Colorado Health Sciences Center and his colleagues at the University of Pittsburgh School of Medicine were recruiting volunteers to join their national weight-control registry for a formal study of how people lost weight and kept it off. They asked me to share my list of reader names, which I was happy to do (participation was voluntary) and I then proceeded to write about what I had learned about our *Eating Well* readers in a story published in January 1996.

What struck me about the letters was that so many people traced their success to a moment of truth, or an epiphany of sorts, that inspired them to finally take charge and *just do it*. One year later, when the formal research study was published in the *American Journal of Clinical Nutrition*, Hill and his team reported the same thing—a full 75 percent of the participants said that they had experienced a moment of truth. There were other striking similarities between what I had found in our decidedly unscientific study and what the researchers found. I will give you the highlights based on the journal report, because Hill's team studied a much larger group in a more scientific manner.

Who and how much. The weight losses of the 784 men and women who contributed to the study were substantial: The average was 66 pounds, and each person had maintained a weight loss of at least 30 pounds for five years. And these people were not amateur dieters—before they had finally succeeded, they had each lost an average of 270 pounds over years of losing and regaining weight. Genetics seemed to play a strong hand: 70 percent had been obese since childhood, and 73 percent had at least one obese parent.

Success triggers. Almost 77 percent traced their success to a specific event, such as being hurt by a negative remark or facing a medical problem, such as type 2 diabetes, arthritis, or heart disease. One woman was inspired to lose weight by making a deal with her daughter to finish college. For others, simply looking at a photograph or in the mirror brought the moment of truth.

Controlling calories in.   People used various methods to keep the weight off, but the researchers did find some common strategies for controlling food intake. The most popular was to limit certain kinds of foods in the diet (92 percent), whereas about a third of the group said they counted either calories or grams of fat. Although all managed to reduce the amount of food they were taking in, they ate nearly five times a day, suggesting that small, frequent meals help with weight control. They also ate most meals at home, averaging less than one meal a week in a fast-food restaurant.

Increasing calories out.   On the calorie-burning side of the equation, virtually everyone exercised to keep their weight down. And not just a little: More than half the participants exceeded the recommended level for losing weight set by the American College of Sports Medicine—one thousand calories per week or approximately thirty minutes of daily walking— by expending two thousand or more calories per week.

Bottom line.   Most of the people had not just put on a few pounds during middle age and then took it off; for them, weight control was a lifelong battle and in part a struggle against nature. The common threads were that they were committed to a lifestyle change and in it for the long haul.

♥

CHAPTER 4

On the Move

Exercise fights insulin resistance. But winning this battle does not necessarily mean you have to become a marathon runner or go to a health club
and wear spandex. Yet this is what many people think of as exercise, which
is a big reason they don't do it: Exercise just seems too hard. Besides, who
has the time?

Take heart. Each time you move, you are fighting insulin resistance.
Muscles are insulin's biggest target; and the more they're used, the more
efficient they become at allowing insulin to supply the glucose they need.
Never mind the fancy clothes, the drive to the gym, and all the other obsta-
cles; what you really have to do is resolve to move more each day.

But don't make the mistake of underestimating how critical it is to be
consistent. The experts tell us that regular, moderate exercise increases
insulin sensitivity but that this effect may be lost within two to three days
of inactivity. Exercise makes insulin work better immediately, even without
weight loss. For example, in one study, insulin resistance was reduced by
58 percent in African-American women who exercised seven days in a row
and whose weight stayed the same. Other studies have shown that the
weight loss that comes with exercising over longer periods of time has
additional effects on insulin resistance, because it lowers body fat. And
exercise should be a family affair: Research suggests it helps improve

insulin sensitivity and ward off type 2 diabetes in young people who have inherited the tendency for the disease.

HOW MUCH IS ENOUGH?

The latest exercise recommendations from the surgeon general and the American College of Sports Medicine are for gentler, yet more consistent exercise—about thirty minutes of moderate physical activity on most, if not all, days of the week. According to extensive research, this amount of exercise is enough to lower the risk of chronic disease. (The old recommendation was for more vigorous exercise for at least twenty minutes three times a week.) To lose weight and lower insulin resistance, it would be even better to go up to forty-five minutes of walking a day. This is a personal decision based on what you can do. Thirty minutes of deliberate aerobic exercise is the minimum; and if you have increased your other activities as suggested in Chapter 3, this may be enough. (Although walking is the most practical aerobic exercise for most people, there are alternatives. See page 35.)

Studies of the effect of exercise on insulin resistance suggest that people who have impaired glucose tolerance and high insulin levels can benefit greatly from the effects of exercise. For example, the type of exercise in the study involving insulin-resistant African-American women showed dramatic results in just one week. Their exercise routine consisted of ten minutes of gentle stretching, thirty minutes of walking on a treadmill, five minutes of rest, and then another twenty minutes of either walking on a treadmill or riding a stationary bike. This total of fifty minutes of walking helped with insulin resistance over the short period of one week. In another study, extremely overweight pregnant women lowered their risk of gestational diabetes (often a warning sign of developing type 2 diabetes later in life) by walking thirty minutes to an hour a couple of times a week.

So exercise fights insulin resistance in more ways than one. There's the immediate effect of improved insulin sensitivity in working muscles, and then there's the long-term effect of helping insulin work better through loss of extra body fat. (You also burn more calories for twenty-four hours after you exercise.) Regular exercise also makes your muscles grow larger (increases lean body mass); and muscles are the biggest users of energy, insulin, and glucose. And study after study shows that being more active is really the only way to keep weight off once you lose it.

There are no two ways about it: You will not be able to keep weight off and lower insulin resistance without becoming more active. Cutting down on calories is only half of the balancing act; burning more calories is the other.

GETTING STARTED

The first and most important step toward becoming more fit is to figure out ways of incorporating extra movement into your everyday life, keeping in mind that you don't have to become an Olympic athlete to lose body fat. Once the plan becomes a habit, you may find you want more because you know how good it makes you look and feel. This is a sign that you might enjoy trying a new active sport or perhaps an exercise class. But always keep in mind that your thirty-minute minimum is your maintenance plan for life. This is what really matters; exercise classes and softball seasons eventually end, but your exercise shouldn't. You can sustain the thirty-minute plan indefinitely, and this is exactly what you need to keep your weight down and your insulin working as well as it possibly can. Let's get started.

Step 1. Get the go-ahead from your doctor. The American Diabetes Association recommends a stress test for everyone over the age of thirty-five years to screen for heart problems. If you have back or joint problems, ask for a referral to a physical therapist. Take his or her advice seriously—physical therapists are highly trained professionals who can help you with particular problems that might keep you from pursuing the exercise you really need. People taking oral medications or insulin must monitor their blood glucose response to exercise.

Step 2. Without changing your daily routine, take a good, hard look at how many minutes you actually move during an average day. Get a notebook, write down the date, and record the number of minutes you actually stand and move your body. Vacuuming, gardening, shopping, and preparing meals count; but leaning against a wall waiting for a bus doesn't.

Step 3. At the end of the day, take some time to add up the minutes. Don't be discouraged if you find there haven't been many. Unless you have already made a concerted effort to move more, it will seem that life just gets in the way. Think about it—commuting, your job, talking on the phone, the television, the computer, heating up a frozen meal in the microwave, and reading the newspaper do not require much physical effort. Did you know that between 1956 and 1990, modern conveniences have reduced our estimated average caloric expenditure by a whopping 65 percent? No wonder weight control is a national problem.

Step 4. Now write down some ideas for fitting in some extra movement during the day. Be creative, and list every possibility you can think of. Look at your notes on how you spend your time to come up with the possibilities—waiting for your ride to work, for example, might be an opportunity to walk to the end of the block and be picked up at a different spot. If you need inspiration, see "Moving Target" (opposite) for ideas. With the eventual goal of walking thirty minutes each day, find one ten-minute time period to start. This will be your minimum daily goal for the first week.

Step 5. Decide how you are going to keep track of your progress. A monthly planner or notebook works well; if you're monitoring your blood glucose, keep the two records together. Review your progress at the end of the week. If there were days that you missed, think about what happened to prevent you from taking your walk, and come up with plan B for fitting it in. Write down how you feel and what your goals are for the coming week. If ten minutes of walking feels like enough, stay with this level until you are ready to move on. If it feels good, set your goal a little higher; it could be twelve, fifteen, twenty, or the full thirty minutes—the important thing is to set a goal you can consistently meet. (You can always go a little farther on a beautiful day when you're feeling great.)

No matter how many weeks or months it takes, the goal is to train your body and your mind to get into that thirty-minute-a-day habit; it could well be the most important thing you ever do.

MOVING TARGET

Work break. It's a great opportunity to kill two (or more) birds with one stone. If you normally go and sit somewhere with the temptation of doughnuts or a vending machine nearby, this is a great time to go out for a walk instead. You can always have a healthy snack at your desk. If you work near a shopping center, you could also get some errands done. If you work in a building in the middle of nowhere (like I do), a walk can be a chance to daydream or enjoy nature (a great stress reducer); or bring a friend along and catch up on the office gossip. Two fifteen-minute walks or three ten-minute walks add up to thirty minutes.

Shop walking. This is a great way to combine exercise with errands or, in the case of recreational shoppers, with pleasure. This strategy is similar to mall walking, in which people who live in cold or dangerous areas go to an indoor mall to exercise. Most malls open early to accommodate walkers. Shop walking can be an occasional way to exercise; a person who usually walks on lunch breaks at work might try it on a Saturday and do some shopping at the same time. The trick is to get in a total of thirty minutes of brisk walking in between stops.

Early bird routines. Are you a morning person, who wakes up bright-eyed, bushy-tailed, and ready to boogie? (Skip this if it doesn't sound like you.) People who get out to walk before everyone else's day begins have the advantage of getting a jump on their day both mentally and physically. Some people find this works for them in the summer when the sun comes up early; they switch their routine as the days grow shorter.

Television time. Viewing time can be converted to walking time. Not that you have to go cold turkey, but are those *Seinfeld* reruns really that funny the third time around? Watch less television, and use the time to take your walk. Or have your cake and eat it too: Walk and watch television at the same time. A treadmill might be a big investment, but it is well worth it if you make up your mind to use it.

> **Travel walking.** Here's a great way to keep up your exercise when you're away from home, and there are several kinds. There are the walks people take when they go on business trips, which simply involve putting on comfortable shoes, going out the hotel door, and exploring a city on foot. There is also the not-so-much-fun kind of walk you take in the airport while you wait for your flight to leave. And then there's the best kind of travel walk, the kind you take on vacation. Plan your own walking vacation or talk to your travel agent about the many organized walking and hiking tours that are now available.

FINDING THE TIME

Not having enough time is the most common reason people give for not exercising. This was once an obstacle in my mind, too; but the real reason was that I didn't make exercise a big enough priority. Besides, I knew I couldn't be a marathon runner like some of my friends. Interestingly, it was working with people with type 2 diabetes that made me finally get out and exercise.

I was working as a research dietitian on a study of the effects of exercise and diet on type 2 diabetes. My job was to help the study volunteers follow a diet, while one of the doctors supervised their exercise program at the university gym. As I met with the volunteers, they kept on telling me how much they were enjoying their exercise, and a few suggested that I go over and walk with them. Their enthusiasm made me realize that lack of time was only an excuse. And as I saw how much each person was improving, I came to understand that it's really important to compare yourself only to yourself: The comparison that matters is between the out-of-shape person you once were and the fitter person you have become. Everyone, whether she's nineteen or ninety, stands to benefit from regular exercise. So more than fifteen years ago, I started out walking with the study volunteers; and though I sometimes enjoy other types of exercise, such as aerobic dance, my daily thirty-minute walk is my mainstay.

This is not to say that time isn't an issue with three children and a full-time job (and a book to write). On many days I think I'm going to get out at lunchtime, but meetings and work get in the way. But as soon as I see an opportunity, I change my shoes and go out the door. If the entire afternoon goes by and I don't get out, I have stopping points on my way home from work where I park my car, walk for 30 minutes, hop back in, and continue home.

If you have a boss who doesn't believe in breaks, be diplomatic and tell her that you are under doctor's orders to take exercise breaks during the day. (I know doctors who write prescription walk breaks for people who have difficult bosses.) Of course, there will be days when everything works against your walk, so if you've given it an honest try, tomorrow's another day. But make sure you put yourself first: You are your number one priority, so there really shouldn't be very many days when other people's needs can't wait while you get your exercise.

WALKING TIPS

The one thing you really need is comfortable shoes. All of your good intentions could be ruined if you start out walking too far in a pair of floppy old loafers and end up with blisters and aching feet. Do they have to be expensive walking shoes? Not necessarily, but shoes designed for walking may very well be the best because they are made with extra support and cushioning. There are many different types of walking shoes available and each one fits a little differently; some are good for people with a high instep, others work for wide or narrow feet, still others are more comfortable for flat feet. Some people find that running or hiking shoes work better for them. The point is, you need to find the pair that feels right, so take a couple of hours and try on different shoes. And while you're at it, buy yourself a couple of pairs of thick, cushiony socks.

Other than making sure your feet feel good, all you need to do is exercise a bit of common sense. Avoid extreme heat or cold, inspect your feet daily, and don't exercise when you are sick. If you're taking drugs to lower glucose, always keep a snack or packet of glucose in your pocket in case of hypoglycemia.

Loose layers of comfortable clothing will allow you to take off a jacket and tie it around your waist if you get too hot. In cool weather a windbreaker with a hood is ideal because it is light and warm; if it gets cold, the hood can keep you warm by preventing heat loss from the top of your head. A windbreaker with zippered pockets can also hold your car keys, sunglasses, lip balm, or whatever else you might need. I usually wear my office clothes to save time, add a windbreaker (and maybe a sweater), change my shoes, and go.

OTHER TYPES OF EXERCISE

Walking is a form of aerobics, or endurance exercise, the type of exercise that burns calories and makes your heart stronger. Strength training and stretching make your muscles larger, stronger, and more flexible. Although aerobic exercise is the best type of exercise for improving insulin sensitivity, working on strength and flexibility for a few minutes each day is the icing on the cake.

Flexibility is the ability to freely move your joints through a wide range of motion without pain. Gently stretching the muscles surrounding each joint on a regular basis will help improve flexibility and prevent injury. The key is to make sure the stretch is gentle and comfortable; it is not safe to stretch to the point of pain. If you have old injuries or physical limitations, consult with a physical therapist about the best stretches for you. If you don't have problems, refer to a good basic exercise book, such as the *American College of Sports Medicine Fitness Book,* for a simple stretching routine.

The other type of exercise that gives you a big payback for the amount of time it takes is strength training. Consult with a physical therapist or exercise physiologist about the best strengthening exercises for you. Spending just a few minutes two or three times a week for simple weight lifting is enough to make muscles grow larger and stronger. Preserving muscle strength is one of the best ways to fight disabilities and stay independent as we age. And because muscle tissue is such a big user of insulin, bigger muscles also mean better insulin sensitivity. When you increase your muscle mass through strength training and other forms of exercise, your body burns more calories even at rest, because it takes more calories to maintain muscle than fat. Now that's something you can really look forward to!

VARIETY IS THE SPICE OF LIFE

What if walking is not possible because of bad knees, extreme hot or cold weather, or lack of a safe place to walk? If you have access to a pool, you might think about swimming. Not exactly a duck in water? Don't worry; the worst swimmers actually get the best workouts. Water offers a lot of resistance, so flailing about and inefficient swim strokes produce a greater challenge to your heart and lungs. The net result is not only an aerobic workout but strength and flexibility training as well.

You might also try stationary cycling, a type of exercise that has worked very well for me lately. Living in Vermont and working long days that are short on daylight have moved my exercise sessions indoors during most of the work week. At a yard sale I spent $25 on a stationary bike that retails for $450. I think the person who sold the bike probably didn't know the key to success with home exercise equipment. The trick is to set yourself to do another activity while pedaling. Let's face it: No one can stand the boredom of staring at the wall and puffing away for very long. But if you get into a routine of watching a favorite show on television, reading, or listening to tapes as you pedal, you are far more likely to look forward to and stick with your daily exercise routine. I actually reviewed this book while riding on my stationary cycle!

The bottom line for weight and blood glucose control is finding ways to exercise that are doable on a daily basis. Start out slowly and gradually increase the intensity and length of your workout sessions. And mix it up! As long as you stick with your daily time commitment, you can walk, pedal, swim, row, dance—cross-training is good for you!

—ROBIN EDELMAN,
Registered Dietitian, Certified Diabetes Educator, and Exercise Enthusiast

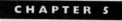

CHAPTER 5

The Good Fat Diet

The ideal diet for type 2 diabetes allows you to control your blood sugar and lose weight, lowers your risk of heart disease, *and* makes you happy because the food tastes good. The Good Fat Diet can help you achieve all of these goals. The purpose of this book is to share with you the science behind this diet and give you all the practical information you need to bring it to the table. But before you go on, remember that exercise is equally important for your overall health, even though many more pages of this book are devoted to how you eat. It just happens that with nutrition, there's much more explaining to do.

You also have to be clear about the reasons for taking on the considerable work of changing your lifestyle: To avoid an early death from heart attack or stroke; to keep type 2 diabetes disease from progressing to the point at which you have to take insulin; and if heart disease doesn't get you first, to avoid blindness, kidney failure, and amputation. The alternative is to look and feel better, not in the least because you will have overcome the combined effects of genetics and environment by the sheer force of your own will.

TWO MODELS OF HEALTHY EATING

Much of the information we have about how diet can support health and longevity comes from research comparing eating patterns in different parts of the world. After learning how our energy-dense food supply and our sedentary lifestyle encourage diet-related diseases, it should come as no surprise that the two best models of healthy eating come from areas of the world where people do not live in this way.

The Seven Countries Study, completed in the 1960s and the best and biggest study of this kind, found the two healthiest diets to be in the Mediterranean and in parts of Asia. What was amazing was that these two diets were radically different in the amount of fat they contained. The Asian diet was very low in fat, whereas the Mediterranean diet was fairly high in fat. At first researchers were puzzled by this difference, because at the time they were studying this information, it was thought that all high-fat diets were bad. But as they studied the diets more closely, they made some very important observations. Most of the fat in the Mediterranean diet was coming from olive oil, a monounsaturated fat; and like the Asian diets, it was very low in *saturated* fat. The diet data told researchers that wherever saturated fat intake was low, people had less heart disease. On the other hand, heart disease was rampant wherever saturated fat intake was very high, namely in Finland, the United States, and the United Kingdom. Many studies since have supported the finding that saturated fat is the single biggest culprit in raising the bad (LDL) cholesterol in the blood.

At the time the information was collected, processed foods were virtually unavailable in Asia and the Mediterranean. People relied on what they could grow or catch in their native surroundings, and the bulk of their calories came from whatever was most abundant—in Asia, where vast expanses of land were devoted to growing grains, it was rice and wheat; in the Mediterranean, where olive trees had been cultivated for centuries, it was olive oil. (Back in the United States, hamburgers and fries were fast becoming staples.)

So here were two very healthy eating patterns, both low in saturated fat, both low in processed foods. But they also had something else in common that made them protect against diet-related diseases. Both the Asian and the Mediterranean diets are plant based (lots of grains, fruits, and vegetables; only a little meat and dairy products), which means they are rich in dietary fiber as well as antioxidants and other protective natural chemicals. In Asia, for example, a typical meal consisted of several large bowls of rice, a variety of vegetables, tofu, and small amounts of dried fish. A typical Mediterranean meal might consist of a large plate of fresh greens and tomatoes dressed with olive oil and lemon juice, and a plate of pasta with olive oil and beans, or maybe eggplant tossed with tomato sauce and a little cheese.

Which would you choose? If you love Italian and Greek food, you're in luck. It turns out that although both diets help prevent diet-related diseases, once you have type 2 diabetes, there are more reasons to choose a Mediterranean-type diet, not in the least of which is the food. It's easy to love.

THE SEVEN COUNTRIES STUDY AND THE MEDITERRANEAN STORY

When traveling through southern Italy in the early 1950s, medical researcher Ancel Keys was impressed with the quality of the local food. Long before such ideas were commonplace, he speculated that the eating patterns were related to the low rates of heart disease in the region. When he got back to the States, Keys assembled a distinguished group of scientists to examine diet and disease patterns around the world. Household by household, they painstakingly gathered dietary information on thirteen thousand people in sixteen population samples in seven countries (Italy, Greece, Finland, the Netherlands, Yugoslavia, Japan, and the United States). In 1970, the results from the Seven Countries Study established a clear link between saturated fat intake, blood cholesterol, and heart disease.

Yet it would take almost another twenty years to complete the analysis of the data and for the details of the Mediterranean diet to come to light. In Crete, where men often downed a glass of olive oil before going out to the fields for the day, the consumption of total fat was near 40 percent of calories, higher than any other country studied; still, Cretan men lived the longest. The fact that olive oil is very rich in monounsaturated fats eventually led to more studies and the conclusion that monounsaturated fat is indeed a safe fat. And we now know that the other components of the traditional Mediterranean diet help protect against not only heart disease but cancer and type 2 diabetes as well.

HOW TO EAT LIKE A MEDITERRANEAN

Olive oil. The main source of fat consumed for centuries throughout the Mediterranean is now recognized as an ideal source of fat for maintaining heart health. Olive oil is used in cooking and to dress fresh vegetables.

Beans, beans, beans. Because of their high protein content, beans and other legumes are the "poor man's meat" of the Mediterranean. Compared to juicy steaks and hamburgers, they are far healthier choices, because they are rich in fiber and other protective substances. Lentils, broad beans, chickpeas, and white and red kidney beans are commonly served with grains, greens, and pasta or simply dressed with olive oil, a little vinegar or lemon juice, garlic, and herbs.

Greens, greens, greens. One of the eating habits in Italy that impressed Keys was the variety of greens eaten each day. In fact, this is such a tradition that there's even a word for eating greens: *mangiafolia*. Green leafy vegetables are a gold mine of protective plant substances, including omega-3 fatty acids (page 64), folate, beta-carotene, and other important carotenoids.

Nuts, more good fats. Archaeological excavations suggest that ancient civilizations relied on nuts as a staple food, even before cereal grains. Widely used in Mediterranean cooking, almonds, walnuts, chestnuts, and pistachios add protein, good fats, vitamins, minerals, phytochemicals, and rich, wonderful flavor. Nuts—walnuts in particular—are another plant source of omega-3 fatty acids.

Great grains. Bulgur, bread, pasta, couscous, cornmeal, polenta, rice, oats, and barley—a Mediterranean meal never is without at least one grain or grain product. Grains are rich in complex carbohydrates, vitamins, minerals, and fiber.

> **Wine.** Moderate drinking is well-documented as protective against heart disease. And—now for the *really* good news—research also suggests that alcohol improves insulin resistance (page 87). This does not mean that people who don't drink should start; but drinking wine with meals, the pattern in Mediterranean and the healthy way of imbibing, can be part of a healthy diet.

FAT-FREE VERSUS SAFE FAT

Back to the United States. In the 1980s, while researchers were still working out the details of the different types of fat and how they affect disease risk, Americans began to focus on one fact: Fat makes you fat. By the early 1990s, fat-free and reduced-fat foods began flooding the market, and many Americans became obsessed with the idea that all fat is bad. But like most things in life, the answer is not that simple.

After several years of snacking on fat-free treats, Americans are fatter than ever. The problem is that it is too easy to overdo it with fat-free ice cream, cookies, and other treats; and many people do by overlooking the fact that fat-free is not necessarily calorie-free. Another explanation for this phenomenon comes from research. Study after study has shown that people simply eat more to make up the calories when they're offered fat-free refined foods instead of the regular-fat versions. And while it is certainly true that fat calories contribute to weight gain, a highly refined diet also contains excess calories from concentrated carbohydrates and protein.

The somewhat surprising lesson learned from this nationwide experiment is that fat or no fat, refined foods are a source of extra calories; yet when they do contain fat, they're more satisfying. This suggests that trying to eliminate fat is not the best way to lose weight, particularly when you want an eating plan that is satisfying and that you can be on for the rest of your life. In fact, preliminary results from an ongoing Boston study at Brigham and Women's Hospital led by Dr. Frank Sacks and registered dietitian Kathy McMannus suggest that people lose weight just as well on a high-monounsaturated-fat diet as they do on a low-fat diet. But as shown by other studies, the high-monounsaturated diet is better for the blood cholesterol profile, blood sugar, and triglycerides.

A Mediterranean-style diet containing a moderate amount of safe fats and lots of unrefined high-fiber foods fits the bill for fighting all diet-related diseases, particularly type 2 diabetes. It makes far more sense for you to spend your calories on a plate of fresh greens dressed with a little olive oil, rather than on a few fat-free cookies. Containing little more than refined sugars and flour, the cookies will raise your blood sugar and most likely your triglycerides. The fat-containing meal will do neither, and just think about which of these two choices will make you feel fuller and more satisfied. (Not to mention which is more nutritious.)

Thanks to Keys and the Seven Countries Study, we have valuable information about a time when most Mediterranean peoples followed ancient eating patterns and how healthy they were for it. But now their diet is rapidly changing. Just as we have seen elsewhere, people are slowly abandoning their traditional eating habits for the diet of the industrialized world. And as they do, heart disease, cancer, and type 2 diabetes are on the rise.

BRINGING THE MEDITERRANEAN DIET HOME

A strong motivation for writing this book is to help keep the principles of the Mediterranean diet alive for people with type 2 diabetes. But my belief that this approach is better than lower-fat traditional diets, such as the Asian diet or the desert diet of the Native Americans, did not develop overnight; it evolved over a twenty-year career of planning, researching, and writing about diets. I am convinced that this model of healthy eating makes sense not only for diabetes but for lowering the risk of *all* diet-related diseases.

As a nutritionist, my interest in type 2 diabetes began in the early 1980s when I worked as a research dietitian. The focus of many of our studies was insulin resistance, obesity, and type 2 diabetes. To make a long story short, among the important lessons I learned was that restricting calories can make people lose weight temporarily no matter what diet you use. And believe me, I have seen them all: the all-meat diet (protein-sparing-modified-fast), the all-liquid diets (Cambridge diet), and other forms of very low calorie torture. But as soon as people went off these bizarre regimens, they would put the weight back on with a vengeance. I learned that there is only one way to keep weight off: Replace refined foods with unrefined foods and become more active on a daily basis.

When I went on to pursue my interests in teaching and writing at *Eating Well* magazine, a whole new world opened up for me—food as pleasure, and not just as a dietary prescription. It was through the magazine that I discovered the food of the Mediterranean and through a series of wonderful seminars sponsored by a group called Oldways (page 85) that I was introduced to the science supporting the benefits of this diet.

But my conversion to the Mediterranean way did not evolve in a vacuum. I, too, was once caught up in the fat-free fervor that swept the rest of the country. My husband has a strong family history of heart disease, so at home we were very careful to limit fat. I also taught people to recognize the hidden fat in foods to help them lose weight and lower their cholesterol. However, the more I learned about the research that had begun with the Seven Countries Study—and the more I learned about the food—the more I began to adopt the Mediterranean diet principles in my own life. Soon, my family was eating more and more vegetable, bean, and pasta dishes and sticking completely with olive oil. (I even use light olive oil for baking.)

I also found myself mentioning the Mediterranean diet in the nutrition classes I teach for heart patients. But when the results of the Lyon Diet Heart Study came out in 1994, it became more than a mention. You better believe I began telling my students how the Mediterranean diet could help protect them against second heart attacks. And because my cardiac rehabilitation groups always include people with type 2 diabetes, I began to realize how *very well* this diet fits the needs of people trying to control their blood sugars.

BUT WILL IT PLAY IN PEORIA?

If you're worried that you will have to become a gourmet cook to be on this diet, don't be. The best diet for diabetes is based on principles learned from the Mediterranean example, but this does not mean you have to eat exactly the way they did on Crete in the 1960s. (And you

THE LYON DIET HEART STUDY

The results of the Lyon Diet Heart Study were nothing short of amazing. Survivors of heart attacks who followed a Mediterranean-style diet rather than the usual American Heart Association (AHA) diet were more than 70 percent less likely to suffer a second heart attack or death from cardiovascular disease. Not only do these results support population studies that find the Mediterranean diet to be protective, they show the impact people can make on their own health by eating their own food in their own homes. And more than anything else, it shows that the Mediterranean diet is doable. The people in the study were given an initial one-hour diet instruction by a research dietitian and a cardiologist. *Just one hour.*

The five-year study, which began in Lyon, France, in 1990, included 605 people who had already suffered heart attacks. The volunteers were divided into two groups: a Mediterranean diet group and an AHA diet group. The Mediterranean diet plan was quite simple: more vegetables, more legumes, more grains, more fish; less meat; not a day without fruit; and no butter and cream. The only fats allowed were olive oil for cooking and a special high-monounsaturated-fat spread, which was supplied to the volunteers and their families. The AHA diet plan focused on limiting total fat to 30 percent and saturated fat to 10 percent of calories, with no emphasis on monounsaturated fat.

In an average follow-up period of a little over two years, there were sixteen fatal heart attacks and seventeen nonfatal heart attacks among the 289 people on the AHA diet, compared to three deaths and five nonfatal heart attacks among the 295 people on the Mediterranean diet. (Of the 605 volunteers who entered the study, 21 had dropped out.) When the researchers analyzed the volunteers' diets, it was found that both groups were eating around 30 percent of their calories from fat. The main difference was the type of fat: According to analyses of the volunteers' blood, the AHA group had consumed more polyunsaturated fatty acids, and the Mediterranean group had consumed more monounsaturated and omega-3 fatty acids. (For the researchers' ideas on how the diet worked, see page 66.)

definitely won't be starting off your day with a glass of olive oil.) Believe me, no one loves true Mediterranean food more than I do; but I simply do not have the time to cook that way very often, and I don't expect that you do either. Besides, many authentic dishes call for olive oil by the cup, and none of us can afford that many calories. The Good Fat Diet is a calorie-controlled Mediterranean-style plan; and although many of my recipes were inspired by the real thing, they are not necessarily authentic. But they are easy.

For example, most serious cooks prepare bean dishes from scratch with dried beans; but I say, why go through all that soaking and cooking when the soluble fiber in canned beans lowers blood sugar just as well? Not to mention the fact that canned beans come out perfect every time so you don't have to worry about ending up with hard beans or bean mush. In fact, I am not ashamed to admit that my cupboard is loaded with canned beans, tomatoes, and dried pasta—my dietary staples.

The ingredients are also not limited to foods native to the Mediterranean. As far as health is concerned, we can learn from the example of eating a diet rich in soluble fiber and monounsaturated fat, and then add other foods that give us similar benefits. For example, black beans, native to South America, and oats and rye grown in colder climates are also rich in soluble fiber, so why not also use them to lower blood sugar and cholesterol? And don't forget peanuts, one of America's contributions to our Mediterranean-style eating plan.

As a matter of fact, the ingredients for the recipes and meal plans in this book can be found in any supermarket. The most abundant food supply in the world gives us the good along with the bad, so let's take advantage of the great ingredients and products, such as prepared salsa, turkey cutlets, and low-fat dairy products. The point is to learn from the Mediterranean example, not be a slave to it; the diet only improves by expanding the variety of foods and adopting it to your own needs.

A Mediterranean meal can be as simple as a large platter of fresh greens or roasted vegetables, chopped nuts, olive oil, balsamic vinegar, a little feta cheese, and some crusty whole-grain bread. A conventional low-fat version of this meal would leave out the cheese, nuts, and oil and probably make up the calories with white bread, lean meat, and maybe some fat-free cookies. But what about the effect on blood sugar? Think about it. With a diet rich in fruits, vegetables, and grains, there's room for a little cheese, oil, and nuts; and it is still possible to lose weight. In fact, the combination of lots of fiber and reasonable amounts of fat will make it easier to lose weight, because you will feel satisfied. Just make sure you stick with the good fats and plenty of soluble fiber to control your blood sugar and help protect your heart.

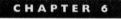

CHAPTER 6

Count On Fiber

One of the best ways to keep foods low in calories and more satisfying is to leave them alone. Foods in their natural state contain fiber, the parts of plants that are virtually calorie free because we can't digest them. Fiber slows you down when you eat because it makes you chew, fills you up, and holds many times its weight in water. Of course, we are talking only about foods from plant sources here; animal products do not contain fiber.

Eating more dietary fiber works toward the main objective of controlling type 2 diabetes: losing weight to lower blood sugar. In fact, eating enough fiber is essential to weight control for everyone, because foods naturally high in fiber are the opposite of foods high in calories: You might say they are energy dilute instead of energy dense. For example, 4½ slices of whole wheat bread have about the same number of calories as ½ cup of Ben & Jerry's butter pecan ice cream. The bread, however, takes up more space and is certainly more filling.

Experts recommend 25 to 35 grams of dietary fiber a day; the average American eats less than half that amount.

The typical industrialized diet is very low in fiber. Refining raw foods like wheat, sugar cane, corn, and soybeans removes the indigestible fiber to get white flour, sugar, corn syrup, corn oil, and soybean oil. This is not *always* a bad thing—getting rid of what you have to chew is a good idea if you want to feed a starving person, because it allows you to pack in a lot of calories into, say, an 8-ounce can.

HIGHLY REFINED FOODS ARE OKAY FOR PEOPLE WHO NEED *MORE* CALORIES

Liquid meals in a can, such as Ensure and Sustacal, are good examples of highly refined foods that were originally developed to feed people who were starving and too sick to eat. Suggesting that a healthy person eat this way makes many health professionals' skin crawl, but those incredibly irresponsible television ads sure make it sound like a good idea. ("Doctor recommended"? For very ill cancer patients, maybe.) There is absolutely no reason on earth that a healthy person shouldn't get his or her calories in their original, chewable package of fiber, vitamins, minerals, and all the known and yet-to-be-discovered natural chemicals that make food good for you.

But when the vast majority of people are struggling to limit the calories they take in, highly refined foods are a big problem. For example, it's much easier to inhale a sweet, gooey fruit bar rather than fresh fruit because it contains very little of the real thing. A look at the ingredient list of a popular mixed-berry bar shows that the first three ingredients are sugar, high fructose corn syrup (sugar), and corn syrup (more sugar), not to mention partially hydrogenated oil and a considerable list of other refined ingredients. For the 130 calories in one of these bars, you could have ½ cup of fresh blueberries, ½ cup of blackberries, and ½ cup of raspberries—the fruits pictured on the front of the box. You would also get more than 8 grams of dietary fiber, which is 8 grams more than you'd get from the bar.

Refining also removes important nutrients and protective plant chemicals from food, which is another contributing factor to our high rates of chronic diseases. But let's limit our focus now to fiber and take a look at why many experts believe that stripping fiber from the food supply is a big contributor to type 2 diabetes.

SOLUBLE FIBER LOWERS BLOOD GLUCOSE

Since the 1970s, there have been a whole series of studies comparing the blood glucose response to different types of dietary fiber and fiber-containing foods. These studies, done mostly by Canadian and British researchers, have established the fact that restoring fiber to the diet helps control type 2 diabetes. When researchers began feeding people high-fiber and low-fiber meals, they quickly established that soluble fiber slows down the rise of blood glucose after a meal. Soluble fibers form a gel when they meet water, and if you've ever used Metamucil, which is rich in soluble fibers, you've seen this in your glass after you add water. This gel gets in the way of digestion and slows nutrient absorption and thus the rate at which glucose enters the bloodstream.

A good demonstration of soluble fiber slowing things down is a comparison of blood glucose levels after eating a bowl of jelly beans and after eating a bowl of oat bran cereal. Even if you consumed exactly the same amount of carbohydrates, the rise in blood glucose would be lower after the cereal than after the jelly beans because the soluble fiber in the oat bran would get in the way; whereas in the candy there's no fiber to slow things down.

And while we're on the subject, this is exactly what researchers started doing in the late 1970s when the test for blood glucose from a finger prick became available. They tested high-carbohydrate foods—everything from mashed potatoes to ice cream—to compare their effect on blood glucose with the effect of drinking pure glucose. Researchers even came up with a fancy name for it: glycemic index (page 56). What they found was big news at the time: It doesn't matter if the carbohydrate is simple (sugar) or complex (starch), the rise in blood glucose is quite similar, and the big factor limiting the rise in blood glucose is the presence of soluble fiber.

There are several benefits of this effect of soluble fiber. First of all, a meal rich in soluble fiber feels more satisfying for a longer period of time, not only because it really fills you up, but also because it is digested more slowly so you don't get hungry again as quickly. And the research suggests that including soluble fiber in a meal helps avoid hyperglycemia (high blood sugar). Keep in mind, however, that the total rise in blood glucose depends on the composition of a meal as a whole, so the relative proportions of protein and fat also have to be factored in.

Soluble fiber also helps out in the cholesterol department. That lovely gel binds bile acids, which are made and recycled by the liver from blood cholesterol. Bile acids are stored in the gallbladder and are released to emulsify fats during digestion. When the soluble fiber in a meal binds bile acids, it doesn't just slow them down, it carries them out of the body and prevents them from being reabsorbed and reused. Because the liver has to use up more cholesterol to make new bile acids, there is a net decrease in blood cholesterol level. A cholesterol-lowering drug made from soluble fiber, cholestyramine, works exactly this way, and so would Metamucil and similar laxatives if you took them often enough.

OAT BRAN: THE COMEBACK KID

You probably remember all the hoopla about oat bran lowering blood cholesterol. But then there was another study showing that other foods could lower blood cholesterol just as well. Many people saw this as just another flip-flop by scientists, but the truth is that the soluble fiber in oat bran does make a difference. However, because so many other components of the diet can easily confound results, it has been hard to pinpoint exactly what one particular food does or doesn't do.

Nevertheless, a more recent, very carefully controlled study did indeed show a clear benefit in oat bran helping control type 2 diabetes. The study, again Canadian, tested the effect of oat bran bread on blood glucose levels in eight men with type 2 diabetes. For twelve weeks, the men ate a weight-maintenance diet; for four men, the diet included six servings of oat bran bread and for the other men, six servings of white bread. For the next twelve weeks, each group switched to the other type of bread. The men maintained their weight throughout the twenty-four-week study. During the high-fiber periods both blood glucose and insulin response after breakfast were lower, total cholesterol and LDL cholesterol were lower, and the ratio of LDL to HDL was reduced by 24 percent.

This study is important to you because it shows what soluble fiber can do to help control type 2 diabetes. And the effect is separate from fiber's other benefit of helping people feel full while losing weight, which *also* lowers insulin resistance and blood glucose. The men in the study purposely did not lose weight, and still the soluble fiber helped lower the levels of glucose and insulin in their blood. At the same time, the lowering of the ratio of bad to good cholesterol was substantial, and certainly would be expected to lower the men's risk of heart disease if they kept up their fiber intake after the study was over.

But perhaps the most important lesson of this study is that one easy change in eating habits can have a significant impact on health. And switching to a fiber-rich bread is a change that is manageable for everyone (page 97). With the other changes outlined in this book, the improvement would be magnified. The Breakfast Cakes on page 187, which contain 3 grams of soluble fiber (5 grams total fiber) each, are rich in soluble fiber. Consider these types of foods important weapons in the fight against type 2 diabetes and heart disease.

RYE BREAD: THE LATEST STAR

Just after the oat bread study was published, a very different study from a different part of the world also pointed to the beneficial effect of another kind of fiber-rich bread. It was a large Finnish study that analyzed the dietary habits of 21,930 middle-aged men. When all of the risk factors for heart disease were taken in account, the men with the highest fiber intake had a 30 percent lower risk of dying from heart disease than the men with the lowest fiber intake.

That fiber protects against heart disease came as no surprise, but what was interesting is that the researchers were able to pinpoint one particular food—rye bread—as a protective factor. It turns out that the popular whole-grain rye bread is such an important part of the Finnish diet that, on average, men actually get the recommended amount of 25 grams of fiber each day. (American men are lucky if they get half that.) We would all do well to develop such a habit, but we can't depend on most of the light fluffy stuff that passes for bread in this country.

THE OTHER FIBER

Although soluble fiber is known to lower both blood glucose and blood cholesterol, two major health studies involving thousands of people—the Nurses Health Study and the CARDIA Study—have found a strong association between eating insoluble fiber (from cereals and whole grains) and reduced risk of developing type 2 diabetes. So don't underestimate the value of *all* high-fiber foods for fighting type 2 diabetes.

Whole wheat products and wheat bran are the richest sources of insoluble fiber, the type of fiber better known for maintaining regularity and preventing colon cancer. A bread that contains both whole wheat flour and oats or rye gives you the best of both types of fiber. Better yet, take it one step further and choose a bread that combines whole grains and flaxseeds (page 100) for the deluxe health combination. And please note how full you feel after eating a sandwich made with high-fiber, whole-grain bread compared to eating a sandwich made with white fluff. Pay close attention to including fiber in all of your meals and snacks—this is one of the secrets of calorie control.

FIBER-RICH FOODS

FOOD	TOTAL DIETARY FIBER (GRAMS)	SOLUBLE FIBER (GRAMS)
Unprocessed wheat bran (½ cup)	14.0	*
Kellogg's Bran Buds (⅓ cup)	13.0	4.0
Kellogg's All-Bran, extra fiber (⅓ cup)	13.0	*
Kidney beans, canned (1 cup)	7.0	1.0
Quaker Oat Bran Hot Cereal (½ cup dry)	6.0	3.0

FOOD	TOTAL DIETARY FIBER (GRAMS)	SOLUBLE FIBER (GRAMS)
Potato, with skin	5.0	1.2
Pear (1)	5.0	0.7
Rolled oats (½ cup dry)	4.0	2.0
Artichoke (½ cup)	4.0	2.4
Pumpkin, canned (½ cup)	4.0	0.6
Prunes (5)	3.0	1.4
Strawberries (1 cup)	2.8	0.6
Orange (1)	2.2	0.9
Whole wheat bread (1 slice)	2.0	*
Apricots, dried (4)	2.0	0.6
Banana (1)	1.6	0.6

Note: Most other fruits and vegetables contain about 2 grams of total dietary fiber per serving.

Sources: Marlett JA. Content and composition of dietary fiber in 117 frequently consumed foods. *Journal of the American Dietetic Association* 1992;92:175–186; Pennington JAT. *Bowes and Church's Food Values of Portions Commonly Used.* New York: Harper & Row, 1987; manufacturers' food labels.

*Trace Levels.

♡

CHAPTER 7

Common Sense About Carbohydrates

If you have been led to believe that eating sugar causes diabetes, the first thing you need to do is to eliminate this notion from your thinking for good. This common misconception will only get in the way of tackling the real issues. But if you have been blaming sugar and other carbohydrates up until this point, don't feel bad, because there is a long history behind this well-entrenched belief. In ancient times, it was noticed that a condition that caused people to waste away and die was linked to sugar in the urine. (The term *diabetes mellitus* is Latin for "sweet urine.") The mysterious affliction was, of course, type 1 diabetes

We now know that neither type of diabetes is caused by sugar. Type 1 diabetes is an autoimmune disorder in which the body's own immune system attacks and destroys the insulin-producing beta cells of the pancreas. And even though it is clear that type 2 diabetes is an inherited disorder brought to the surface by too many calories and too little activity, there is more confusion than ever about carbohydrates. This chapter will help you sort through the carbohydrate issues.

THE "BREAD IS FATTENING" MYTH

Whenever the topic of weight control comes up, someone inevitably mentions the problem of bread, when, in reality, the only problem with bread is that Americans don't eat enough *good* bread. But the belief that bread makes you fat is deeply entrenched in the American psyche: In a recent Gallup survey, 49.5 percent of overweight shoppers said they believed that bread is fattening; 35 percent of shoppers who were not overweight agreed. Research shows the opposite—eating more bread replaces more calorie-dense foods and helps people lose weight. Overweight college students lost an average of nine pounds when fed eight slices of bread a day for ten weeks. In a similar study, another group of students eating high-fiber bread lost considerably more than a group eating white bread. People with type 2 diabetes can and should enjoy reasonable amounts of good bread, the fiber-rich kind, which helps lower blood glucose, even without weight loss, as was shown in the oat-bran-bread study described in the last chapter.

THE ANTI-CARBOHYDRATE CRAZE

Self-proclaimed experts have been writing best-selling books that blame high-carbohydrate foods for weight gain, insulin resistance, and just about every other health problem known to humankind. But this is entirely untrue. Think about it. You don't have to wear a white lab coat to understand what causes type 2 diabetes. The disease is practically unknown among Asian people who follow traditional very high carbohydrate diets based on wheat or rice. But when Asians come to the United States and start eating double cheeseburgers and sitting in front of the television with the rest of us, they begin to have the same problems with weight, heart disease, and type 2 diabetes. Japanese American men living in Hawaii, for example, are commonly plagued by type 2 diabetes: In the Honolulu Heart Program, 17 percent of men aged seventy-one to ninety-three had diagnosed diabetes, 19 percent had diabetes and didn't know it, and 32 percent had impaired glucose tolerance. The idea that eating carbohydrates causes insulin resistance is utterly false; eating the right kind of carbohydrates actually helps avoid insulin resistance. The problem is that anti-carbohydrate diet books are often best-sellers because people want to believe that eating *more* meat and cream is a good idea. How could this be when heart disease is our number one killer?

THE FAT-FREE MYTH

About seven or eight years ago, food manufacturers began to catch on to what experts were saying about high-fat diets causing heart disease and making us fat. Soon new fat-free and low-fat products began arriving on grocery shelves like nobody's business. Some of those products, such as reduced-fat dairy products, mayonnaise, and leaner meats, have been a true blessing. But other products, namely the reduced-fat desserts and snack foods, appear to have contributed to the country's increasing girth by creating the idea that fat-free means calorie-free. Unfortunately, this problem helped fuel the anti-carbohydrate movement. Yet the bottom line is that treats are treats; and whether they're pure sugar or fat laced with sugar, neither is a good idea when it brings in calories over and above what is spent each day. On the other hand, if you are active and doing well with your diet, there is room for a treat once in a while; but do yourself a favor, go for quality over quantity.

CARB COUNTING

One of the problems of grouping people with type 1 diabetes, who take insulin, with people with type 2 diabetes, who do not take insulin, is that diet education often focuses on learning to count carbs. This is not the most important priority for people with type 2 diabetes. People with type 1 diabetes have to carefully match the grams of carbohydrates they take in over the course of a day with their expected insulin levels, as well as other factors such as exercise. But what is critical for people with type 2 diabetes is calorie control. The way to manage type 2 diabetes is to lower insulin resistance, and the way to lower insulin resistance is to lose body fat and move more on a daily basis. However, as we have seen, the amount of fiber you get along with your carbohydrates is key. If you want to count grams of something, count grams of fiber.

THE GLYCEMIC INDEX

The ideal high-carbohydrate food has not only plenty of satiety value and nutrients but also as little an impact on blood sugar as possible. This is why scientists came up with the **glycemic index,** a way of rating foods according to how fast and how high they raise blood sugar (glycemia: *glyc* = "sugar or glucose"; *emia* = "blood").

When the glycemic indexes of foods were first measured in 1981 by the Canadian research team of David Jenkins and Thomas Wolever, the results were not at all what people expected. Up until that time, it was assumed that starchy, high-complex-carbohydrate foods would not raise blood sugar as much sugary foods, but Jenkins and Wolever found that some starches raise blood sugar almost as much as a load of glucose. Surprisingly, the glycemic response to potatoes and white bread were similar to sweets and sugary cereals. On the other hand, beans, lentils, and dried peas were found to elicit a low glycemic response; pasta and rice were ranked somewhere in between.

After many more studies and much debate, it became clear that the effect of foods on blood sugar depends on many factors. As we have seen, there is the important soluble-fiber effect of slowing carbohydrate absorption rate, which explains why foods like beans and oats have a low glycemic index. And then there is the question of how rapidly a starch can be digested. Starches are called complex carbohydrates because they are made up of many glucose molecules all linked together. The glycemic index studies showed us that the *way* the glucose molecules are linked together determines how fast we can digest them. Some, like potato starch, are so rapidly broken down by digestive enzymes that they cause a rise in blood sugar that is almost indistinguishable from that of pure sugar.

The way a starchy food is prepared also affects how rapidly it is digested and absorbed: Pasta cooked *al dente* (still firm) raises blood sugar more slowly than does overcooked, mushy pasta; mashed potatoes raise blood sugar more rapidly than do cubed and boiled potatoes. To make matters more complicated, subtle differences, such as the ripeness of a banana, can double the glycemic index. Moreover, people don't usually eat just one food at a time, they eat a mix of foods; and the fat content of a meal also slows carbohydrate absorption.

With all of these complicating factors, it's not surprising that the value of teaching people about the glycemic index became a subject of hot debate among diabetes educators. Experts in the United States, led by dietitian Anne Coulston and diabetes researcher Gerald Reaven (who first described insulin resistance syndrome), finally suceeded in keeping the glycemic index from being required in diabetic teaching. They made it clear that it was unnecessary to impose yet another diet worry on people with diabetes, because their blood sugar levels are the sum total of so many factors. (If you are curious about the glycemic index, see "Resources" for how to get a listing of the glycemic indexes of three hundred individual foods.)

Indeed, other research suggests that the insulin response to what we eat is the underlying determinant of blood sugar levels overall. In a nutshell, it appears that diets high in good carbs—those high in fiber—require less insulin to dispose of blood sugar than do those high in the not-so-good carbs. In fact, eating a diet high in cereal fiber (whole grains) has recently been found to protect against both obesity and type 2 diabetes in the CARDIA Study. When researchers tracked changes in fasting insulin levels and body weight in 3,709 adults for a seven-year period, they found a strong association between eating refined carbohydrates and increased weight and fasting insulin.

The findings of the CARDIA Study are consistent with the Nurses Health Study, which found that women who ate the most low-fiber, high-glycemic-index foods, such as white bread, colas, jams, and potatoes had 2½ times the rate of type 2 diabetes as the women who ate the most high-fiber, low-glycemic-index foods.

So it seems that when you look at the big picture, as researchers did in these large health studies involving thousands of people, the way to eat carbohydrates is with as much of their original fiber as possible. Focus on eating carbohydrate foods that contain fiber, and your blood sugar will be all the better for it.

GOOD AND NOT-SO-GOOD CARBS

Just as there are good fats and bad fats, there are good carbs and not-so-good carbs. (They can't be called "bad" because even pure sugar isn't in the same league as pure hydrogenated vegetable shortening in terms of calories and what it does to your arteries.) But there is a big difference between refined and unrefined carbohydrates, the type that helps make the caloric density of the typical American diet even denser. The kinds of foods we tend to gravitate to are often a combination of fat and refined carbohydrates—what are sometimes called the sweet fats and the savory fats. Sweet fats include pies, cookies, ice cream, doughnuts, and candy bars; savory fats include potato chips, corn chips, buttery popcorn, and biscuits, all of which contain saturated fat and/or hydrogenated fats, the artery cloggers. But we love them because during our evolution calories meant survival, and our brains remain programmed to go for the most concentrated forms of energy. But this doesn't mean we can't use other parts of our brain to motivate ourselves to go for less calorie-dense foods, which taste equally good, to go with our less energy-dense lifestyle.

RATING CARBOHYDATES

EXCELLENT CARBS*	OKAY CARBS	NOT-SO-GOOD CARBS
Beans, all kinds	Pasta	Sweets
Whole wheat bread	White rice	White bread
Oatmeal	Potatoes	Chips
Fresh fruit		Sugared soft drinks
Real rye bread		Cookies
Bulgur		Cakes
Whole wheat couscous		Jams and jellies
Tofu		Sugary cereals
Barley		
Whole grains		
Brown rice		
Whole wheat pasta		
Buckwheat		

*Read more about the excellent carbs in "Stocking the Healthy Pantry" on page 96.

NOT-SO-GOOD CARBS VERSUS GOOD FATS

When the research suggested that olive oil is indeed a safe fat to eat in terms of heart disease, scientists became interested in the possibility that replacing some dietary carbohydrates with monounsaturated fat might lead to better diabetes control. Sure enough, when they compared the effects of two diets equal in calories—one higher in monounsaturated fat and the other higher in carbohydrates—in people with type 2 diabetes, they found that blood glucose control was better on the high-monounsaturated-fat diet. The volunteers who ate the monounsaturated fat diet for six weeks also had more desirable levels of LDL cholesterol and triglycerides.

This study and others suggest that as long as you pay attention to calories, you are better off replacing high-carbohydrate foods that are devoid of fiber and nutritional value with monounsaturated fats. The idea that monounsaturated fats can be better for your blood sugar and blood fats than refined carbs probably takes some getting used to because of the myth that all fats are bad. In other words, a few walnuts are better for you than a fat-free snack cake. And on that note, let's move on to learn more about how you can make fats work for you.

♥

CHAPTER 8

Making Fats Work for You

Some people think that the number one diet goal for type 2 diabetes is limiting fat, others think it is limiting carbohydrates. It is neither—limiting calories is most important. But because most calories come from fat and carbohydrate, they should be balanced within that calorie limit to give you the best possible control of your blood sugar and cholesterol. Eating a reasonable number of calories from fat makes sense, because fat does not raise blood sugar. But you must choose your fats wisely: The bad fats contribute to heart disease, whereas the good fats protect against it. This chapter goes over the good guys and the bad guys and just how they earned these reputations.

You have probably heard that fat makes you fat, so you may wonder if it is really possible to eat fat and still lose weight. Eating too much fat certainly can make you fat, but so can eating too much carbohydrate or too much protein. The reason fat has been singled out as such a big villain is that people who eat high-fat, Western-type diets generally suffer from high rates of heart disease, cancer, and obesity. This type of diet contributes to heart disease because it is too high in the bad fats, it contributes to cancer because it is too low in protective fruits and vegetables, and it makes people fat because it is too high in calories from all sources.

It certainly is possible to lose weight while eating a reasonable amount of fat. Studies have shown that people with type 2 diabetes lose weight just as well on higher-fat diets rich in monounsaturated fat as they do on lower-fat diets. But when they are rich in good fats, the higher-fat diets are better at fighting the problems of high blood sugar, low HDL cholesterol, and high triglycerides—not to mention that the diet makes people happier. When researchers ask volunteers which diet they prefer, they usually chose the Mediterranean-type diet over the low-fat diet. And any chef can tell you why: Fat enhances the flavor of food.

FAT 101

The fats in the foods we eat are made up of fatty acids. There are three types of fatty acids—saturated, polyunsaturated, and monounsaturated—and all fats contain a mix of the three. But a fat is referred to as one of these three types, usually according to the type of fatty acid that predominates. Corn oil, for example, is called a polyunsaturated fat because 60 percent of its fatty acids are polyunsaturated. In general, monos and polys lower blood cholesterol when they replace saturated fats in the diet. "Comparison of Dietary Oils" (page 62) shows the proportions of the three types of fatty acids in commonly consumed fats.

THE SAFE FAT: MONOUNSATURATED

Equal in priority to the number of calories you take in and burn each day is the quality of the fat you eat. The fat you add to your food should always be high in monounsaturates. As you can see from the chart on the next page, olive oil is the most monounsaturated oil; and though canola oil comes in second, it is the other smart choice, because it is low in saturated fatty acids and is a source of omega-3 fatty acids, the other kind of good fat. Nut oils (and the nuts they come from) are also rich in monos, but they are not used as much in cooking because they are very expensive.

So why are monos better than polys? Up until a few years ago, people were taught that polyunsaturated fats were the fat of choice because research showed they lowered blood cholesterol when they replaced satu-

Comparison of Dietary Oils

Although we refer to fats as either polyunsaturated, saturated or monounsaturated, all dietary fats are really mixtures of the three types of fatty acids. A fat is usually classified according to the fatty acid that predominates.

Canola oil and olive oil are the safest fats, because they are both low in saturated fatty acids and high in monounsaturated fatty acids.

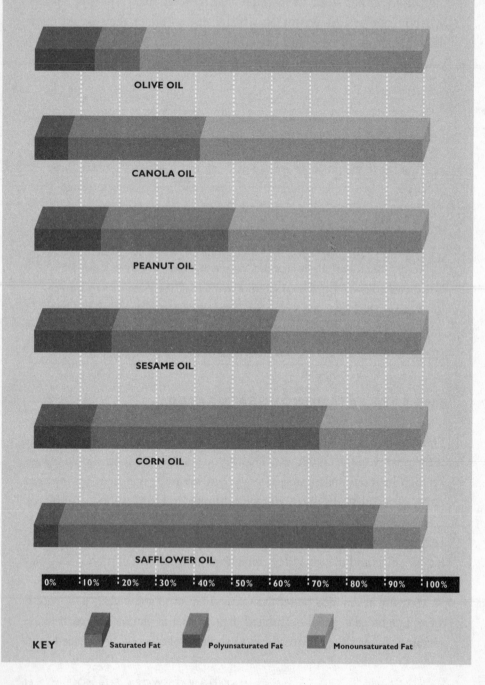

OLIVE OIL

CANOLA OIL

PEANUT OIL

SESAME OIL

CORN OIL

SAFFLOWER OIL

0% 10% 20% 30% 40% 50% 60% 70% 80% 90% 100%

KEY   Saturated Fat   Polyunsaturated Fat   Monounsaturated Fat

rated fats in the diet. Monos were pretty much overlooked, in part because they were thought to be neutral—neither raising nor lowering blood cholesterol—and frankly, because the United States is not a big producer of monounsaturated oils. Olive and canola oils were almost exclusively imported products—olive from the Mediterranean and canola from Canada. Because soybeans and corn are big crops in the United States, we consume a lot of soybean and corn oil.

But when the information about the Mediterranean diet began to trickle down to clinical research (where diets are tested on people in a controlled setting), researchers began looking more closely at the effects of monounsaturated fats. And when they did, it became clear that replacing saturated with monounsaturated fat is every bit as effective for lowering blood cholesterol as replacing them with polys.

So now there were two types of low-saturated- fat diets that would lower blood cholesterol: one high in polys and one high in monos. And there was also the third type of low-saturated-fat diet: the very low fat diet, in which all fats are low and the majority of calories come from carbohydrates (the Asian diet model). Of course, by then, researchers knew that total cholesterol wasn't the whole story, so they began to look at how the three diets affected the good (HDL) and bad (LDL) cholesterols. Sure enough, monos lowered the bad without lowering the good, whereas the high-poly and high-carb diets both lowered the good along with the bad. This fact is extremely important for people with type 2 diabetes, because low HDL cholesterol often goes along with insulin resistance. And low HDLs are a powerful predictor of heart disease.

Eating monos instead of polys may offer additional protection for your heart, because monos are more resistant to oxidation. Polys are easily oxidized; and as they are shuttled along in the blood on lipoproteins, they make the entire lipoprotein vulnerable to oxidation. And when the bad lipoproteins—the LDLs—become oxidized, they become the most artery-clogging kind (page 14).

EVER WONDER WHAT A "CANOLA" IS?

Actually, there's no such thing as a canola plant; canola oil is pressed from rapeseed, the seed of a variety of mustard plant. But because of obvious PR problems, a Canadian producer renamed the oil: can for "Canada" and ol for "oil."

The bottom line is that the other two diets often used to protect against heart disease—the high-poly diet and the very low fat diet—are not the best choices for people with type 2 diabetes. And even though they lower the bad cholesterol, they have not been shown to protect people who already have heart disease from having a heart attack.

THE OMEGA-3S: A LITTLE HELP FROM YOUR FRIENDS

The omega-3 fatty acids are the other kind of fat that works to protect you against things that go wrong in type 2 diabetes. To begin, researchers think that the reduction in heart attacks in the Lyon Diet Heart Study came largely from the omega-3 fatty acids in the Mediterranean diet and their ability to reduce cardiac arrhythmias and blood clotting. This effect has also been shown in studies that have examined diets high in fish and fish oils, which are rich sources of omega-3s.

FIVE REASONS TO LOVE MONOS

Monos are good for your blood sugar.

Monos are good for maintaining HDLs.

Monos are good for lowering LDLs.

Monos are good for lowering triglycerides.

Monos resist oxidation.

Research on the effects of omega-3 fatty acids is relatively new, but it is fast becoming an area of intense study, because they are believed to have far-reaching benefits to health. Some of the interest has stemmed from the studies of fish oils and heart health and from the finding that an omega-3 fatty acid called docosohexanoic acid (DHA) is critical to brain development and brain function. The body makes DHA from the parent of all omega-3s—alpha-linolenic acid, an essential nutrient that originates in plants. Fish and other animals that feed on wild plants also make DHA; and when we eat these animals, we get ready-made DHA. This means that a person who is a strict vegetarian needs to get alpha-linolenic acid to make DHA from plant foods such as greens, legumes, nuts, and seeds.

To keep things simple—and to avoid using long chemical names like docosohexanoic, alpha-linolenic, and worse—let's simply use the term *omega-3s,* because from now on it will work just as well. All you have to remember is that there are plant omega-3s and there are animal omega-3s, the kind that fish, humans, and other animals make from plant omega-3s.

One of the problems with our modern diet, according to many

researchers, is that it is far lower in omega-3s than the diet consumed throughout human evolution. The foods we eat today are much higher in omega-6 fatty acids, the kind that predominate in polyunsaturated vegetable oils. At one time, we ate more omega-3-rich plants that grew in the wild and omega-3-rich meat from animals that foraged on wild plants. But with modern agriculture, we now have mass production of foods that are poor in omega-3s, such as the corn we feed our livestock and many of our vegetable oils. This is why fish has now become such an important source of omega-3s; luckily they still feed on omega-3-rich plankton and not on corn.

Among the researchers who believe that our low intake of omega-3s contributes to many modern health problems is Dr. Artemis Simopoulos, who chaired the nutrition coordinating committee at the National Institutes of Health for nine years. In her excellent book written for consumers, *The Omega Diet*, she says that at one time the ratio of our intake of omega-6s to omega-3s was less than four to one; but in modern times, the ratio can be as high as twenty to one.

This altered ratio can lead to both physical and mental problems. Because of the brain's need for omega-3s, low levels may contribute to depression, attention-deficit hyperactivity disorder, and violent behavior. It is beyond the scope of this book to describe all of the health problems that are suspected of being linked to the twenty-to-one ratio; suffice it to say that many are related to the fact that the two kinds of omega fatty acids compete for the same enzymes, which transform the fatty acids into substances that have profound effects throughout the body, including blood clotting, heart rhythm, and immune function.

There is, however, one connection that is very important for people with type 2 diabetes. Although the research is quite new, it appears that diets low in omega-3s may contribute to insulin resistance. When researchers make laboratory animals insulin resistant by feeding them diets high in saturated fats and omega-6 fatty acids, they can normalize them by feeding them omega-3s. According to Simopoulus, this may work because of the way omega-3s affect insulin sensitivity at the cellular level. Cell membranes, made largely of fatty acids, are a direct reflection of the kinds of fatty acids in the diet. When cell membranes are rich in omega-3s, they become very fluid with greater numbers of and more responsive insulin receptors. When the diet is poor in omega-3s, cell membranes are also poor in omega-3s, which may make them insulin resistant.

Australian researcher Dr. Leonard Storlien found that people whose muscle cells have a particularly high ratio of omega-6s to omega-3s are more likely to be insulin resistant and obese. Interestingly, Storlien has also found that Pima Indians, who have the highest rates of insulin resistance in the world (page 5), have much lower levels of omega-3s in their muscle cells than other people eating a similar diet. He suspects this may be caused by a genetic glitch that makes it difficult to get omega-3s incorporated into cell membranes. Theoretically, this problem may be one cause of the stubborn insulin resistance that plagues the Pimas.

When you take this new research into consideration, keep in mind that even without the insulin resistance connection, study after study has shown omega-3s to be powerful protection against death by heart attack. Other research suggests that omega-3s are a valuable ally in the war against cancer: both for prevention and for boosting the effectiveness of traditional therapies aimed at keeping existing cancers from spreading. Low levels of omega-3s are also being investigated as causes of autoimmune diseases, such as asthma, type 1 diabetes, rheumatoid arthritis, ulcerative colitis, lupus, and psoriasis. For more information, I recommend Simopoulus's book and her Web site for updates on omega-3 research (see "Resources").

Omega-3s in the Diet

In traditional Mediterranean diets, people ate fish whenever it was available, but they also ate lots of green leafy vegetables and nuts, the plant sources of omega-3s. The people eating the Mediterranean-type diet in the Lyon Diet Heart Study were also getting a good amount of omega-3s; but ironically, they were from canola oil, a relatively new type of oil not available in traditional Mediterranean diets. This came about because some people enrolled in the study didn't want to be limited to olive oil and wanted something they could spread on their bread, so the researchers came up with a canola oil spread. It turns out that this was a valuable addition to the diet because not only is canola oil high in monounsaturates, it's a good source of plant omega-3s.

After all was said and done, the levels of omega-3s in the blood samples of the Lyon volunteers were as high as those in blood samples from the men on Crete, who were studied in the Seven Countries Study back in the 1960s. No doubt the men on the island ate more wild greens and fish than did the people in the French study, who ate canola oil. But you don't have to live in France or Greece to change the ratio of omega-6s to omega-3s in your diet. You can start today with one well-planned trip to the supermarket.

FIVE WAYS TO CHANGE YOUR OMEGA-6 TO OMEGA-3 RATIO FOR THE BETTER

1. Avoid oils that are rich in omega-6s, namely those that are highest in polyunsaturates: sunflower, corn, safflower, and grapeseed oils.

2. Use olive and canola oils as the main sources of fat in your diet. They are also high in monounsaturated fats (technically omega-9s), which have their own benefits and will help tip the omega-6 to omega-3 ratio in the right direction.

3. Eat seafood as often as possible. All seafood, including shellfish, have some omega-3s, but the most concentrated sources are the fatty fishes such as salmon.

4. Eat walnuts, greens, and legumes on a regular basis. Walnuts are a good source of omega-3s; and although greens and legumes contain smaller amounts, they're kind of like exercise: Getting them every day will make a significant difference in the long run.

5. Consider adding flaxseeds or flaxseed oil to your diet, particularly if you are a vegetarian or if you don't like fish. See page 100 to find out how.

NOTE: These strategies have been incorporated into the meal plans (Chapter 12).

BEST SOURCES OF OMEGA-3S

FOODS	TOTAL OMEGA-3 FATTY ACIDS (GRAMS)
Flaxseed oil, 1 tablespoon	7.0
Sardines, 3½ ounces	3.0
Mackerel, 3½ ounces	2.5
Flaxseeds, ground, 1 tablespoon*	2.0
Herring, 3½ ounces	1.7
Salmon, 3½ ounces	1.4
Canola oil, 1 tablespoon	1.5
Walnut oil, 1 tablespoon	1.2
Walnuts, chopped, 1 tablespoon	0.7
Tuna, albacore, 3½ ounces†	0.6–2.1

Note: *Fruits and vegetables, particularly greens, are also sources of omega-3s, and although the amount they contain is low, eating the recommended 5 to 10 servings a day adds up.*

*Don't eat more than 3 tablespoons of raw flaxseeds a day. They contain a substance that interferes with the body's use of iodine, which can increase your risk of goiter.

†The omega-3 content of canned albacore tuna depends on its total fat content, which varies from 1 to 7 grams per serving because the fat content of tuna varies according to the age of the fish and the time of year it was caught. Check the manufacturer's label; the higher the total fat, the higher the omega-3s.

MINIMIZE THE NEGATIVE

And now for the fats to avoid: saturated fats from full-fat dairy products and meat, hydrogenated fats from processed foods, and highly polyunsaturated oils. Eating too much saturated fats is probably the worst thing you can do. Not only are they bad for your heart but there is evidence that they also may be involved in insulin resistance, because saturated fats cause insulin levels to remain high after a meal.

Now, the reality is that you will get small amounts of saturated fat from certain high-protein foods in your diet, such as chicken, reduced-fat dairy products, and lean meats; but the benefits of these foods will outweigh this drawback, as long as you keep your serving sizes to the amount given in the plan. The idea is to balance the fats in the diet to keep the bad fats as low as possible and the good fats as high as possible.

The other way bad fats sneak into the diet is through the hydrogenated fats in processed foods. Don't let this happen: Whenever you see the word *hydrogenated* on an ingredient list, substitute the word *saturated* in your mind, because hydrogenated fats are artificially saturated. The process of hydrogenation creates trans fats as a by-product, and they also raise blood cholesterol and have recently been linked to breast cancer risk. (Monos and omega-3s have been associated with low rates of breast cancer.) Here's where quality-control really counts: Food labels are not required to list the amount of trans fats in foods, so you have to look at the ingredient list. The closer partially hydrogenated oil or fat is to the top of the list, the more of it the product contains, because labels list ingredients in order by weight. (And don't be fooled by the word *partially*—it most definitely doesn't mean that it's only a little bad for you.) Hydrogenated fats and fiber-depleted carbohydrates are usually found in the same products, and these are the ones to avoid as much as possible if you want to protect your arteries *and* your blood sugar.

ACCENTUATE THE POSITIVE

Within your fat and calorie limit, you should focus on eating monunsaturated- and omega-3-containing fats. What this means in terms of shopping and cooking is keeping the good fats on hand and reading the ingredient lists on food labels to avoid the bad fats. (Throw out that old bottle of corn oil; it's prone to oxidization because it is high in polys, so it's probably already rancid.) Thankfully, there are more and more prepared foods with good ingredients, because many people are willing to pay a little more for the convenience. In Chapter 10, I will tell you how to find these products and suggest some of the best prepared foods that are currently on the market. I'll also tell you how to stock your pantry—and your briefcase—with quick-and-easy foods that will help you keep the good fats up and the bad fats down.

THE GOOD FATS	THE NOT-SO-GREAT FATS*	THE BAD FATS
Avocados	Corn oil	Coconut oil
Canola oil	Grapeseed oil	Dairy fat
Fish fat	Soybean oil	Hydrogenated oils
Flaxseeds	Safflower oil	Meat fat
Flaxseed oil	Sunflower oil	Palm oil
Nuts		Palm kernel oil
Nut oils		
Olive oil		
Olives		
Peanut butter		
Peanuts		

*These fats should be consumed in moderation, because they are high in omega-6s and raise the ratio of omega-6s to omega-3s in the diet.

♥

CHAPTER 9

What You Need to Know About Supplements

Every time you pick up a newspaper there seems to be news about dietary supplements fighting one disease or another. At the same time, the official stand of most health groups is that supplements are not necessary if you eat a balanced diet. Should you be taking supplements? If so, which ones?

Unfortunately, the supplement information that people really need to help improve their health is clouded by several issues. One is that the term *dietary supplement* can legally be used to refer to just about anything that can be packed into a pill or potion. Another is that the multi-billion-dollar supplement industry often takes bits of scientific research and stretches the truth to make unfounded health claims. On the other hand, when there is real evidence that a supplement might actually provide health benefits, the experts are held back from coming out and making recommendations until there are enough studies to be absolutely sure that a particular supplement is safe and effective. But the truth is, science has a long way to go before we'll have a complete understanding of human nutrition and the levels of nutrients (and other phytochemicals) needed for optimal health.

The best example of a supplement that may very well make a big difference in your health is vitamin E. Yes, even though what you've heard about vitamin E sounds too good to be true (usually when supplement claims sound too good to be true, it's because they're not true), most of what you've heard is probably accurate. Taking large doses of vitamin E appears to offer protection against heart disease, boost the immune system, and delay the progression of Alzheimer's disease. But the results of the long-term studies needed to give the official go-ahead for people to start taking vitamin E in large doses are not in yet. Still, the benefits certainly seem to outweigh the risks, so much so that most cardiologists support their patients who take vitamin E, as long as they are not taking other drugs that might make it inadvisable. There is also reason to believe that vitamin E may be of particular benefit to people with diabetes.

While vitamin E is the star in terms of real, scientifically explained benefits, the supplement shelves are filled with useless, expensive, and possibly harmful pills that you're better off without. Yet aside from vitamin E, and possibly calcium, chromium, and vitamin C, there is a very important supplement with a list of scientifically proven benefits that are just too good to ignore. It's also cheap, safe, and available at any supermarket: the all-around multi-vitamin-mineral supplement. And although supplements will never take the place of a real food, in this chapter we will review the benefits of these useful adjuncts to a healthy diet.

THE GOOD NEWS ABOUT VITAMIN E

You have probably heard about vitamin E and heart disease because it has been the subject of extensive research over the past several years. You may have also heard that this antioxidant vitamin can boost the immune system, delay the progression of Alzheimer's disease, and possibly lower the risk of prostate cancer. These findings are all legitimate, but compared to the heart disease research they are still very preliminary. If for no other reason, people with type 2 diabetes stand to benefit from vitamin E because they are two to five times as likely to have heart disease as everyone else. But there's more. Other studies suggest that vitamin E helps with several problems associated with type 2 diabetes.

Let's start with heart disease. It was not until the early 1990s that scientists from several areas of study began to piece together a new understanding of how cholesterol in the blood damages artery walls. First one clue and then another led them to discover that LDLs—the bad cholesterol—are even worse for arteries when they are oxidized (page 14). In fact, it looks as if it may be the damage caused by oxidized LDLs that starts off the process of atherosclerosis in the first place.

Over the past several years, there has been a lot of excitement about this cardioprotective effect of vitamin E. In addition to experiments showing that vitamin E does indeed reduce LDL oxidation, men and women who took vitamin E on their own and were followed for more than a decade had a 40 percent lower risk of heart disease. Other studies showed that people who supplemented their diets with vitamin E after cardiac bypass surgery or balloon angioplasties did significantly better than those who did not. The amount of vitamin E needed for this protection is thought to be at least ten times the current recommended amount. At high levels, vitamin E reduces blood clotting by making platelets less sticky, which gives additional protection against heart attack and stroke.

Here's the really good news: People with diabetes may stand to benefit even more than others from extra vitamin E. Some researchers think that one reason type 2 diabetes heightens the risk of heart disease is that high blood sugar makes oxidation more of a problem than it is when blood sugar stays in the normal range. Indeed, blood from people with diabetes contains more oxidized fats, possibly because high blood glucose sets off oxidation reactions; and people with diabetes have been found to have lower levels of protective antioxidants. Research does suggest that vitamin E protects LDLs from oxidation in people with type 2 diabetes.

Vitamin E may also help with the long-term complications of diabetes, because it prevents oxidative damage to the cells in the eyes and kidneys. In a recent Boston study, researchers found that large doses of vitamin E normalized blood flow problems in the retina and improved kidney function in patients with type 1 diabetes.

WHY YOU SHOULD TAKE A MULTIPLE SUPPLEMENT

Most health professionals, myself included, were taught that people don't need to take extra vitamins if they eat a balanced diet. This may be true for the person in perfect health who eats the perfect diet and who knows he's inherited a perfect set of genes with no tendencies for heart disease, diabetes, or cancer. I personally take a daily multiple supplement. And so do most health professionals I know. This is not to say that any supplement can lessen the need for any of us to eat well and exercise, but you stand to gain more from one good all-around supplement than a whole health-food store full of unproven pills and potions.

Why? First of all, it is never a good idea to take one nutrient at a time without good reason, as in the case of vitamin E, and possibly vitamin C, chromium, and calcium. Large doses of one vitamin or mineral can affect the absorption of others and may expose you to the risk of consuming toxic amounts. Of course, vitamin manufacturers love it when you buy a bottle of this and a bottle of that, because they can make much more money that way. For pennies a day, a good generic, all-around supplement makes sure you get all the basics in a safe balance. In fact, several of the nutrients found in multiple supplements have been shown to be extremely protective, which gives us at least five good reasons for making them a daily habit.

1. Multis Contain Folate and Friends

Folate, also called folic acid, became an important nutrition concern in the 1990s for two separate but equally important reasons. First, it was found that women who take folate during early pregnancy reduce their risk of having a baby with neural-tube birth defects. Then it also became apparent that folate may have a previously unacknowledged role in helping prevent heart disease. The link is a substance called homocysteine (page 11).

Folate is needed to convert homocysteine to another amino acid, and when the supply is low, homocysteine levels build up in the blood. High levels of homocysteine damage arteries; safe homocysteine levels are linked with adequate folate and lower heart disease risk. Because most Americans do not get the recommended amount, a recent law has mandated the fortification of cereal products with folate. But even with fortification, it is estimated that 76 percent of Americans will still not get 400 micrograms of folate per day, the amount believed to help guard against birth defects and heart disease. Folate is one of the few nutrients that is better absorbed from supplements than it is from food. Most multis provide the amount of folate most people need to keep homocysteine in the normal range, as well as providing vitamin B_6 and vitamin B_{12}, two vitamins that help folate do this job.

2. Multis Contain Vitamin D

Although you probably know that calcium is important for preventing osteoporosis, you may not know that the body needs vitamin D to make use of calcium to build bones. This would not be a problem if everyone lived in a sunny climate and got out in the sun for fifteen minutes every day, because the skin makes vitamin D when exposed to sunlight. It also wouldn't be a problem if people drank milk regularly to meet their calcium needs, and if the milk were reliably fortified with vitamin D. But none of this is the case, and people living in northern latitudes have been shown to lose bone density in the winter. A multiple supplement with the recommended amount of vitamin D allows you to make the most of the calcium you take in and help your bones stay healthy. Too much vitamin D, however, causes bones to lose calcium, so it is wise to limit your extra D to the amount in your multiple supplement. Other research suggests that adequate levels of vitamin D may help protect against osteoarthritis and atherosclerosis and may possibly offer protection against cancers of the colon, breast, and prostate.

3. Multis Contain Vitamin C

It has become clear over recent years that the amount of vitamin C needed for optimum health is higher than the current recommended dietary allowance (RDA) of 60 milligrams. In fact, by the time you are reading this book, the official recommendation may very well have been raised from 60 to 200 milligrams a day. This is good news for people with diabetes, who have probably had higher requirements for vitamin C all along. Because of its role in the formation of collagen, the main protein of connective tissue, vitamin C is thought to help protect against damage to small blood vessels caused by high blood sugar. There is also evidence that vitamin C helps prevent other complications by interfering with the conversion of blood glucose to sorbitol, a sugar alcohol that damages eyes, nerves, and kidneys. Vitamin C has also been shown to interfere with the formation of glycosylated proteins (when excess blood glucose hooks up to proteins), which are also a cause of long-term damage. And last but not least, vitamin C has been shown to improve insulin action and lower blood glucose in people with type 2 diabetes.

4. Multis Contain Magnesium

Low levels of the mineral magnesium are related to hypertension and insulin resistance in general, and as many as 25 percent of people with diabetes (both types) have been reported to have magnesium deficiency. It may be that magnesium spills over into the urine along with glucose when blood glucose is high; but researchers are not sure about this, because normalizing blood glucose doesn't seem to correct magnesium deficiencies. At any rate, getting enough magnesium is extremely important for people with type 2 diabetes, since low levels are linked not only to high blood pressure and insulin resistance but also to cardiac arrhythmias, high blood fats, and delayed release of insulin. The best food sources of magnesium are leafy green vegetables, legumes, nuts, and whole grains—the mainstays of the Good Fat Diet. The extra magnesium in a multiple supplement is added insurance.

5. Multis Contain Vitamin B_{12}

Extra vitamin B_{12} is a good idea, particularly for seniors, because we tend to secrete less stomach acid as we age, and low acidity reduces B_{12} absorption. A B_{12} deficiency can cause serious damage to the nervous system, yet this damage may go undetected because extra folate in the diet masks the symptoms of a B_{12} deficiency. This has become more of a concern lately since the government has mandated that cereals and other grain products be fortified with folate. Taking a daily multiple supplement provides the B_{12} you need to help avoid a hidden B_{12} deficiency; if you're over sixty-five you may even opt for a senior formula that contains higher amounts of B_{12}.

CHOOSING A MULTI-VITAMIN-MINERAL SUPPLEMENT

The best all-around multi-vitamin-mineral supplement you can buy does not have to be expensive. The vitamins and minerals that go into the pills are all manufactured by one or two huge companies, who sell them to packagers. That's right, the vitamins in the pill that costs you a dollar are identical to the ones in the pill that costs five cents. It's like buying a store-brand grocery item that is every bit as good as the brand-name item—only the price and packaging are different. In fact, some of the best buys around are the house brands of supermarkets, drugstores, and chain stores. Unfortunately I can't recommend specific brands, because they vary so much around the country. However, the American Association of Retired Persons (AARP) has good mail-order deals. (See "Resources" for their toll-free number and Web site address.)

What *Shouldn't* Be in Your Supplement

Unless you know you are iron deficient, look for a supplement that *does not contain iron*. Many products come in formulas with and without iron. Adults do not generally need additional iron, because so many foods are fortified with iron; and there are many concerns and unanswered questions about the consequences of getting too much iron, particularly as we grow older. At high levels, iron is a pro-oxidant, and studies have linked high iron stores to an increased risk of cancer. Some but not all studies have found a connection with heart disease. A recent study found that 13 percent of seniors have iron stores that are too high, whereas only 1 percent were too low. And the only way to rid the body of excess iron is through blood loss.

The other things you don't want in your multi are vague unspecified ingredients like "herbal blends," because this description doesn't tell you anything. Manufacturers use this as a ploy to make people think they're getting something worth paying more money for. Often these supplements are worthless because they are incomplete and don't contain what you really need, like folate and vitamin B_{12}. They may contain something you don't need, like toxic levels of vitamin D. Researchers at a osteoporosis clinic found that several of their patients were suffering from vitamin D intoxication because they were taking products containing unspecified "organ extracts," which turned out to be desiccated animal liver, a concentrated source of vitamin D. This was really unfortunate, because toxic levels of vitamin D weakens bones, the opposite of what it does at the recommended level.

So don't waste your money. Buy a generic multi-vitamin-mineral supplement that contains a balance of real nutrients. See the chart on the next page for what *should* be in a good multiple supplement.

CHOOSING A MULTI-VITAMIN-MINERAL SUPPLEMENT

NUTRIENT	PERCENT DAILY VALUE (OR USRDA)
Vitamin A (as beta-carotene, or as acetate and beta-carotene)	100
Vitamin C*	100*
Vitamin D	100
Vitamin E	100
Thiamin (B_1)	100
Riboflavin (B_2)	100
Niacin	100
Vitamin B_6	100
Folic acid (folate)	100
Vitamin B_{12}†	100†
Pantothenic acid	100
Copper	100
Magnesium	100
Selenium	100
Zinc	100

*At the time this book went to press, the Daily Value for vitamin C was still 60 milligrams, although research suggests that the optimal value is 200 milligrams. Look for a multi that contains 200 milligrams or consider taking a separate tab of vitamin C (page 80).

†Some senior formulas contain extra vitamin B_{12} because older people often have reduced stomach acid secretion, which makes it more difficult to absorb vitamin B_{12}. This might be a good idea if you're over sixty-five or if you know you have this problem.

How much of each nutrient? Only consider products that list the amounts in percent of the USRDA or DV (Daily Value). This will tell you how the amount of a particular nutrient included in the supplement compares to the current official recommendation. Don't buy products that list nutrients only in units like milligrams (mg), micrograms (mcg), and international units (IU), because you have no way of knowing whether the amount is high or low when you can't compare it to the recommended amount. Products that are labeled this way are often loaded with stuff you don't need because, obviously, there are no recommended amounts; and if the pill does contain any real nutrients, you can bet they're not all there in the balance you need.

Other minerals. Some supplements also contain the minerals calcium, potassium, iodine, chloride, and manganese in less than 100% of the DV. These are minerals the body does need, but they are not necessarily included in supplements because they are fairly easy to get from food and because they are needed in such large amounts that the vitamin pill would be too big to swallow if they were all there in the recommended amount. Although it doesn't hurt to have any of these, don't worry if they're not included.

EXTRA SUPPLEMENTS OF CALCIUM, VITAMIN E, VITAMIN C, AND CHROMIUM

The question of whether or not to take other supplements is bound to come up sooner or later. Check with your doctor, diabetes educator, or registered dietitian about taking anything other than a multi-vitamin-mineral supplement. From what we know about nutrients and disease, the four types of single supplements that may do you some good are calcium, vitamin E, vitamin C, and chromium.

Women *and men* who don't include dairy products in their diets should take a separate calcium supplement to help prevent osteoporosis. There is also good evidence that calcium is important for controlling blood pressure; however, the studies that have shown a relation between calcium and lower blood pressure (page 84) have all looked at food sources of calcium. It is not known whether calcium from supplements has the same effect, so it is better to get your calcium from your diet if you possibly can. Calcium from supplements *has* been shown to help protect against osteoporosis.

Even if the multiple supplement contains calcium, it is usually only a small amount, because the full amount would make your vitamin as big as a horse pill. Besides, the best way to absorb calcium is to take it in three separate doses. Look for a calcium supplement that provides 33 percent of the Daily Value in one tablet and take one with breakfast, lunch, and dinner. Don't buy the kind of calcium supplements made from dolomite—the calcium in them is not well absorbed, and dolomite is sometimes contaminated with lead, mercury, and arsenic. Again, make sure you are taking your multiple supplement with 100 percent of the Daily Value for vitamin D, which the body needs to properly use calcium.

Until we have the results of long-term clinical trials, there is no official recommendation for vitamin E; studies have shown heart disease protection from doses of 100 to 800 IU, but many studies have used a dose of 400 IU, which many experts believe is a good level for people at risk for heart disease. The only known risk of taking large doses of vitamin E is associated with its blood-thinning effect, which may increase the risk of hemorrhagic stroke. In this kind of stroke, there is bleeding into the brain that could be caused by or worsened with high levels of vitamin E. This same blood-thinning effect, however, may be how vitamin E protects against the other more common kind of stroke—thrombotic stroke, caused by a blood clot lodged in the brain. In view of vitamin E's substantial benefits and the fact that people have been taking it in large doses for at least twenty-five years with no reported side effects, the risks appear to be minimal. But be sure to talk it over with your doctor, especially if you are taking any blood-thinning medications.

Extra vitamin C may not be as important if you have a multiple supplement that contains 200 milligrams (333 percent of current Daily Value) or if you have an excellent diet. Vitamin C is, however, extremely safe and people with diabetes may have increased needs for extra antioxidant protection, so it might be wise to give yourself the benefit of added insurance. Buy tablets that contain 200 to 250 milligrams, break them in half, and take one in the morning and one at night. This way you should have plenty of vitamin C in your blood to protect against oxidation twenty-four hours a day.

Unlike vitamin E, which is fat soluble, vitamin C is water soluble, and whenever there is too much in the blood it spills over into the urine. Thus vitamin C is an example of when a little is good, more is not better. It is known that around 200 milligrams a day is the level at which the blood and tissues contain all the vitamin C they can hold. Taking much higher levels, such as 1 gram (1,000 milligrams) or more each day, makes the kidneys work harder, which is not a good idea for people with diabetes whose kidneys may already be taxed. The kidneys filter excess sugar out of the blood, and adding to this burden may add to the risk of kidney failure, one of the long-term complications of diabetes. Too much vitamin C can also cause inaccurate blood glucose readings and gastrointestinal irritation.

The trace mineral chromium may be particularly important to people with impaired glucose tolerance or type 2 diabetes because chromium is an essential helper (cofactor) to insulin. And although there is no doubt that a chromium deficiency will cause insulin resistance, whether people with type 2 diabetes are likely to be chromium deficient is very controversial. Unlike magnesium and calcium, minerals the body needs in relatively large amounts, chromium is needed in extremely tiny (trace) amounts; so tiny in fact, that it is almost impossible to determine who has enough and who doesn't. Some researchers believe that people with type 2 diabetes have low levels and that giving them extra chromium improves their insulin sensitivity. Indeed, in a recent study done in China by Richard Anderson from the U.S. Department of Agriculture (USDA), chromium supplementation resulted in dramatic improvements in volunteers with type 2 diabetes. But critics say that the volunteers were probably chromium deficient to begin with, because their food was grown on chromium-depleted Chinese soils.

Yet other research is beginning to support Anderson's contention that chromium supplements may overcome insulin resistance. Diabetes researcher Dr. William Cefalu at the University of Vermont, who is currently conducting a chromium study, believes that there is enough evidence to recommend 400–600 micrograms of chromium a day to his patients with type 2 diabetes. The form of chromium that both he and Anderson say is well absorbed is chromium picolinate. Chromium supplementation is not currently endorsed by the American Diabetes Association because the research is still in progress, so it remains an issue to be discussed with your doctor.

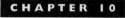

CHAPTER 10

♥

Putting It All Together

Although everything we've reviewed so far may seem scientific and a little overwhelming, a healthy lifestyle really isn't that complicated. In fact, it is surprisingly simple when you are born into that environment. Consider the description of life in rural Italy, from a wonderful book about the food of Liguria by Fred Plotkin:

> It should not surprise you then that in Italy, where people have one of the longest life expectancies in the world, no one lives longer than Ligurians. . . . If you look at Liguria and its people, you will understand. . . . The topography of the place means there is a lot of exertion required: climbing hills and trails, walking up and down steps in cities, tilling terraces carved from the hillside, working aboard ships and boats. . . . The presence of older people is more a part of the landscape in Liguria than it is elsewhere. But these are not feeble old people. A lifetime of work and the Ligurian diet has produced old people who can carry six liters of water up a hundred steps. . . . There is almost no butter and cream in the food and very little cheese. Olive oil and garlic, essential in cooking farther south in Italy, are consumed each day.

Most of us were not lucky enough to be born into such a health-sustaining environment, but we can certainly learn from the Mediterranean example and work on creating our own healthy way of living. Instead of thinking of a diet as something you go on (and then go off), begin thinking of the word *diet* according to its original meaning, "a way of living." The best diet for type 2 diabetes is a pattern of healthy eating *and* becoming more active for life.

If the changes are to be permanent, it is extremely important for you to choose foods and activities you enjoy. This book gives examples of how it can be done with the Good Fat Diet based on the Mediterranean diet model, which is ideal for managing type 2 diabetes and heart disease for two very good reasons: Solid science supports it in every aspect, and the food is good.

I would also like to point out that the Mediterranean diet is anything but a passing fad. The eating pattern not only has supported health and longevity for centuries but also is a perfect match for the new nutrition guidelines from the American Diabetes Association (ADA), which recognizes the value of monounsaturated fats for people with diabetes. And although the ADA does not limit people to Italian or Greek food, this type of eating pattern can bring the dry nutrition guidelines to life. Wouldn't you prefer thinking about eating eggplant Parmesan and pears baked in Madiera, rather than monounsaturated fats, phytochemicals, and dietary fiber?

The good fat meal plans and recipes in the next chapters are based on all of the nutrition stategies for fighting type 2 diabetes and heart disease that have been reviewed in this book. And because hypertension is a big problem that often goes along with both, the Good Fat Diet is also designed with blood pressure contol in mind. In fact, it is really based on two eating patterns. One is obviously the Mediterranean diet model; the other is the DASH diet, an eating pattern that has been shown to be ideal for lowering blood pressure. In this chapter I will explain how these two patterns fit together, review the pros and cons of moderate drinking, and sum up the goals of the Good Fat Diet.

THE DASH DIET

The Dietary Approaches to Stop Hypertension (DASH) diet was developed to lower blood pressure in a study involving 459 people at six major medical centers. And it's not the same no-added-salt routine. In fact, it was what the volunteers ate, and not what they didn't eat, that lowered their blood pressures.

What they did eat were fruits, vegetables, and low-fat dairy products—and plenty of them. The DASH diet contains about twice the amount of fruits, vegetables, and dairy products as the typical American diet and less than half the amount of saturated fat. The effect of this combination was compared to two other eating patterns, one that included the same amount of fruits and vegetables but no dairy products and a control diet that was high in saturated fat and low in fruits, vegetables, and dairy products. The two fruit- and vegetable-rich diets began lowering blood pressure within two weeks, but the diet that included low-fat dairy products lowered it the most.

The volunteers included healthy men and women from various ethnic backgrounds who had normal or slightly elevated blood pressure. The diet was slightly more effective among African Americans and other minority groups who have a high risk of hypertension; however, it lowered blood pressure across the board in all groups regardless of age, gender, or ethnicity. And although the food for the study was carefully planned and prepared in research kitchens, you can get the same benefit at home using the good fat meal plans, which were made to be as similar to the fruit-vegetable-dairy combination diet as possible.

How did the DASH diet lower blood pressure? The researchers suggest several possibilities. First, saturated fat was lower on the DASH diet than in the control diet (7 versus 16 percent), suggesting that eating less bad fat helps lower blood pressure. The salt level was not a factor, because all three diets were carefully controlled to be equal in sodium; however, the DASH diet was rich in potassium, magnesium, and calcium, the three minerals believed to help lower blood pressure.

The DASH study showed what eating fruits, vegetables, and low-fat dairy products can do. And these results were obtained in people with normal or mildly elevated blood pressure, which made the improvement even more significant. In diet studies, it is much easier to show a change in people who already have very high blood pressure or cholesterol, and much harder to show a change in people who don't have as much room for improvement. Yet even though the researchers kept the volunteers from losing weight (the best way to lower blood pressure) and kept the salt intake the same in all groups, they were able to show that the kinds of foods people eat can lower blood pressure. Think what this type of diet could do for your blood pressure when you are also watching calories and exercising to lose weight.

THE OLDWAYS MEDITERRANEAN DIET PYRAMID

A good way to sum up everything good about the Mediterranean diet is to take a look at the Mediterranean Diet Pyramid developed by Oldways Preservation & Exchange Trust. As I mentioned before, I want to thank and give credit to the people at Oldways, who, true to their name, are working to preserve traditional ways of eating in a world of fast food and slow bodies.

THE TRADITIONAL HEALTHY MEDITERRANEAN DIET PYRAMID

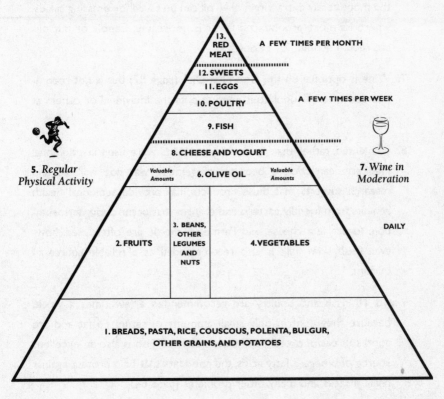

13. RED MEAT — A FEW TIMES PER MONTH

12. SWEETS

11. EGGS

10. POULTRY — A FEW TIMES PER WEEK

9. FISH

8. CHEESE AND YOGURT

5. *Regular Physical Activity*

Valuable Amounts — 6. OLIVE OIL — Valuable Amounts

7. *Wine in Moderation*

2. FRUITS

3. BEANS, OTHER LEGUMES AND NUTS

4. VEGETABLES

DAILY

1. BREADS, PASTA, RICE, COUSCOUS, POLENTA, BULGUR, OTHER GRAINS, AND POTATOES

The Pyramid from the Bottom Up

1. The emphasis is on minimally processed whole grains consumed as often as possible.

2 and 4. Choose seasonally fresh and locally grown fruits and vegetables when they are available. Frozen fruits and vegetables, available year-round, are perfectly acceptable and are the closest match to the nutritional value of fresh.

3. Beans, other legumes, and nuts can stand in completely for animal products as protein sources for people who choose to follow a Mediterranean-type vegetarian diet. Rinsed and drained, canned beans are the equivalent of cooked dried beans and are highly recommended for ease of preparation, low cost, and excellent results in most recipes.

5. Regular physical activity—walking and preparing your own food—is an integral part of this way of living.

6. Less-expensive light olive oil is appropriate for sautéing and cooking; the more costly extra-virgin olive oil can be saved for dressing salads, where its more pronounced flavor is noticeable. Canola or nut oils are recommended for baking.

7. Wine is optional on the Good Fat Diet (page 87) but is not recommended when alcohol consumption puts the individual or others at risk.

8. Fermented, rather than fresh, dairy products were used in traditional Mediterranean cooking because refrigeration was not available; and research suggests that these products may provide additional health benefits from friendly bacteria and changes that occur during fermentation. Yogurt, feta cheese, and Parmesan cheese are often used; however, fresh skim milk is also recommended as a reliable source of calcium.

9 and 10. Fish and poultry are recommended a few times a week, because they contain only small amounts of saturated fat and are good sources of protein and trace nutrients. Fish is also an excellent source of omega-3 fatty acids, the good fats that help protect against heart attacks and many other problems (page 64).

11. Eggs may also be eaten a few times a week, because they are low in saturated fat and high in protein and valuable nutrients. A limit of four eggs per week is the recommendation of the American Heart Association.

12. Sweets are limited to a few times a week. According to the nutrition guidelines from the American Diabetes Association, sugar is acceptable in limited amounts. However, homemade sweets using good fats, nuts, and whole grains are strongly recommended over refined, highly processed products.

13. Meat is recommended only a few times a month; however, small amounts may be used more often to add interest and flavor to food. For instance, 1 ounce of ham or reduced-fat sausage in a serving of soup or beans makes perfect sense in terms of flavor and good nutrition.

The Mediterranean pyramid illustrates the overall composition of the Good Fat Diet, but many people with type 2 diabetes also need a structured way to limit calories. The menus in the next chapter are based on 1,500 calories per day and reflect the principles of the Mediterranean model and the DASH diet.

WEIGHING THE BENEFITS AND RISKS OF ALCOHOL

Although there are definite health benefits associated with moderate drinking, health professionals are often reluctant to discuss them because alcohol may raise the risk of breast cancer and because alco-

PRESERVING THE OLD WAYS

Oldways Preservation & Exchange Trust is a nonprofit organization dedicated to promoting healthy, clean foods and encouraging healthy eating. Oldways was founded in 1988 by K. Dun Gifford jointly with the Harvard School of Public Health. They have since sponsored symposia and educational initiatives demonstrating the importance of our agricultural, culinary, and diet legacies and how the lessons of the past can be applied to present-day problems. For more information, write Oldways Preservation & Exchange Trust, 25 First Street, Cambridge, MA 02141.

GOALS OF THE GOOD FAT DIET

REPLACE THE BAD FATS WITH THE GOOD FATS

Eat less meat and fewer processed foods. Eat more fish and more plant-based dishes flavored with olive oil, canola oil, and nuts. Replace full-fat dairy products with reduced-fat dairy products.

EAT MORE FIBER-CONTAINING FOODS

Plan your diet around vegetables, legumes, fruits, and unprocessed grains. Make sure each meal and snack contains fiber so you'll feel more satisfied with fewer calories.

BURN AT LEAST AS MANY CALORIES AS YOU EAT EACH DAY

Limit calories and take an active role in preparing your own food. Work up to thirty minutes of daily exercise and then to forty-five minutes, if possible.

holism is such a health problem in this country. People with diabetes are often discouraged from drinking because alcohol has the potential for causing dangerously low blood sugar (hypoglycemia) in type 1 diabetes; however, when taken with food, alcohol does not pose this risk for people with type 2 diabetes. But there are definite pluses to moderate drinking for people with type 2 diabetes and heart disease *who are not at risk for alcohol abuse,* and this book would be incomplete without a review of the related research.

First of all, there is really no question that one to two drinks a day offers protection against heart disease, and most of this protection comes from alcohol's ability to raise the good HDL cholesterol. Since the 1970s, study after study has reported about a 40 percent reduction in heart disease risk in moderate drinkers compared to abstainers. And surprisingly, there is also research suggesting that calories from alcohol are not readily stored as body fat. This, of course, seems just too good to be true and remains controversial. The fact remains, however, that many major health studies have found that on average, moderate drinkers are consistently thinner than nondrinkers, and alcohol calories do not cause weight gain in carefully controlled diet studies.

But what is most intriguing for people with type 2 diabetes is that alcohol appears to lower insulin resistance. Large health studies have found that regular moderate drinkers have lower fasting insulin levels and less insulin resistance, and the lower fasting insulin is associated with lower heart disease rates. In fact, some researchers go so far as to suggest that alcohol's protection against heart disease comes from its positive effects on insulin resistance. In a study of female identical twins, the addition of one drink a day to the diet of one twin in each pair resulted in a significant reduction in both insulin and glucose levels after a glucose challenge. Moderate alcohol consumption has also been associated with decreased risk of type 2 diabetes in a Harvard health study that tracked the diet and health habits of more than 41,810 men for six years.

When making the decision to drink or not to drink, the key concept is moderation. At levels higher than one or two drinks a day, the health picture changes drastically: blood pressure rises, triglycerides rise, the cholesterol profile worsens, and blood sugar levels become erratic. And there is no doubt that heavy drinkers die younger than the rest of the population, even without taking into account the toll of accidental deaths from drunk driving.

On the other hand, for some people, a glass or two of wine with dinner can add to the enjoyment of a meal while helping to modulate insulin resistance and heart disease risk factors. If you decide this works for you and you are also on a calorie-controlled meal plan, such as the 1,500-calorie meal plans in this book, I recommend that you not subtract other foods and replace them with alcoholic beverages. The reason for this is that you need all of the nutrients provided by the foods on the plan. Another reason is that as mentioned above, the research does suggest that alcohol calories may not need to be counted in the same way as food calories. Some researchers have suggested that this may be because of alcohol's effect on the insulin, the storage hormone. If moderate drinking lowers insulin levels and insulin resistance, it has the potential of helping rather than hindering weight loss.

♥

CHAPTER 11

Menu for Success

Now let's bring the Good Fat Diet to the table. The remainder of the book provides shopping information, meal plans, and recipes to help you devise your own healthy eating pattern. The recipes are based on what I do in my own home for my own family; and my hope is that if they are good enough and easy enough, people who read this book might incorporate some of them into their own lives.

I also hope it is crystal clear that becoming more active is as important as what you eat and that you will combine the two by preparing more of your own food. Not only is this a way of burning a significant number of calories, as we saw on page 22, it is the best way to eat well.

There are really two aspects of this ideal eating pattern: One is the overall goal of achieving and maintaining a healthier weight; the other is continuing to eat well for the rest of your life. The ideal diet is mostly made up of whole foods, or those as close to their original form as possible. I say "mostly" because there are some processed foods that are worth using because of their convenience, flavor, or nutritional quality; and like most aspects of life, it is not necessary to carry things to the extreme. The ideal diet should bring you pleasure, not deprivation.

The recipes given here are not original—few recipes really are—they are my versions of classic combinations that can help you fulfill the nutrition goals put forth in this book. The food is appropriate for your friends and family because what happens to be best for controlling type 2 diabetes happens to be a healthy eating plan for everyone else as well. Besides, what do you think will entice people over for dinner? Hearing that you're on a "diabetic diet" or that you're planning a Mediterranean feast that you would like to share with them?

People's nutritional needs vary mostly in terms of amount. What is appropriate for your teenage son, for example, may very well be twice as much as you need, so a recipe that serves four might end up serving two or three. You will be doing those you love a favor if you prepare food tasty enough to entice them to eat well along with you.

A PLAN THAT WORKS FOR YOU

There are several approaches used to help people lose weight and control their blood sugar; and if you are already on a plan that works for you, by all means, stick with it. The nutrition information in this book can help fine-tune any plan. If you have been recently diagnosed with type 2 diabetes or heart disease, and you are just starting out on your diet, I recommend seeing a dietitian or diabetes educator to talk over your particular situation; and take this book with you. You are in the driver's seat when it comes to your health, but a little drivers' ed can certainly help you get going in the right direction (see "Resources"). If you feel you don't really need extra support right now—say, if you're changing your diet on your own to help prevent heart disease—you can be assured that this is not a fad diet. All of the recipes and meal plans are consistent with the nutrition guidelines of the American Diabetes Association (ADA) and the American Heart Association (AHA). What sets this diet apart is the big emphasis on eating good fats and lots of fiber, which is taking these guidelines to their highest level.

Depending on your particular situation, there are several ways to use the recipes and meal plans in this book. Ideally, I would like everyone to get to the point of enjoying a Mediterranean-type diet the way I do—for the sheer pleasure of eating without worrying about precisely how much. This is a reasonable goal that can be reached when you achieve a healthy weight and being active becomes second nature. But if you have a long way to go, you need more structure right now, which is the reason for providing meal plans, and not just a series of recipes. And there are several ways to approach the goal of adopting the Good Fat Diet, so before you go on, take a moment to decide on the approach that best describes your needs.

ONE STEP AT A TIME

Making small, gradual changes is a reasonable approach for most people. If, for example, you set a series of small goals and give yourself a week or a month to achieve each goal, you should see big improvements over a year. Tackling diet goals one by one improves your long-term success, because you give yourself time to get used to each change before you move on. Taking on too much at one time can make you feel like you're simply following someone else's set of rules, and the danger is that you may feel so overwhelmed that you give up completely. So unless you have reached the point at which you are completely ready for radical change in eating— and even then you have to make the plan your own—it's best to take it one step at a time. "No Small Change" (below) will give you some ideas about the kinds of changes you might make.

NO SMALL CHANGE

Fat-proof your kitchen. Go through your cupboards and refrigerator and get rid of all the bad and not-so-good fats. You'll live a longer, healthier life without the solid vegetable shortening, stick margarine, butter, high-poly oils, and all products high in hydrogenated fats. Replace these fats with olive oil, canola oil, canola oil spread, and cooking spray made with either olive or canola oil.

Make five-a-day your minimum. Knowing that the people who lowered their blood pressure in the DASH study ate ten fruits and vegetables a day makes five seem like an easy goal. If you're already at five, see if you can do better by trying new and different recipes, such as roasted vegetables (page 135) or baked fruit with a yogurt topping (page 202).

Cut down on red meat. If you're a big meat eater, start out by trying some of the recipes that use small amounts of meat, and perhaps set a goal for preparing meat-free meals one or more times a week. Your ultimate goal could be to have red meat less than once a week.

Count grams of fiber. You may have counted grams of fat or grams of carbohydrates in the past, but one of the most useful strategies for weight control is counting grams of fiber. The way I control my caloric intake is to avoid eating meals or snacks that are devoid of fiber; this way I always feel full and I don't have to count calories. (Check out the fiber content of my recipes, and you will see what I mean.) And I shouldn't have to remind you by now, but fiber has the additional benefit of tempering blood sugar and cholesterol.

Try new recipes. When people tell me they can't cook, I think, "They don't try." I know, I was once there. When I was in my early twenties, my cooking skills were limited to scrambled eggs, until a roommate who was tired of doing all the cooking taught me how to make spaghetti sauce. Anyone can cook. You may not be able to cook up a great meal without recipes—that takes practice—but with recipes, you can prepare simple food that tastes good. Remembering what it was like to start from scratch, I have gone to great lengths to make my recipes easy and my instructions clear, so how about setting a goal of trying a certain number of new recipes a week?

THE EXCHANGE PLAN APPROACH

Many people reading this book may already be on an exchange plan, especially those who have been working with a registered dietitian. This system has been widely used to plan diets for more than thirty years. Exchange lists separate foods into six groups; foods within each group have approximately the same amount of carbohydrates, protein, fats, and calories. The idea is to have a set number of exchanges each day that add up to a balanced diet and a certain number of calories. The drawback of traditional exchange plans is that the foods on each list are not equal in terms of fat quality and fiber content, but this can remedied by focusing on the best choices within each group: oatmeal rather than sugary cold cereal, for example. On the plus side, this system can be a useful way of tracking calories, because the number of exchanges are often listed at the end of recipes and on food labels. Exchanges are listed for the recipes in this book so that people using the approach should have no problem fitting new recipes into their existing plans. For more information on the Exchange Lists for Meal Planning, call the American Dietetic Association/National Center for Nutrition at 800-366-1655 or the American Diabetes Association at 800-342-2383.

CARBOHYDRATE COUNTING

Another approach to diets for controlling diabetes is counting grams of carbohydrates. The goal is controlling carbohydrate intake because it is the carbohydrate content of foods that has the greatest effect on blood sugar. This approach is most useful for people with type 1 diabetes, who need to carefully match the amount of carbs they take in with the amount of insulin they take. This approach is also used for type 2 diabetes, particularly by people with uncontrolled blood sugar who can benefit from carefully spreading out their carbohydrate calories throughout the day. The nutritional analysis of each recipe includes the grams of carbohydrates so that people who use this method can continue to count carbs while paying attention to the other critical aspects of their diet: calories, types of fat, and fiber.

THE ALL-OUT APPROACH

If your blood sugar, triglycerides, cholesterol, and blood pressure are all too high and your doctor tells you to lose weight or else, you may be ready to go all out and follow the meal plans as closely as you can. But this is a big commitment, so before you get going, there are two very important considerations. One is that you also need to work on meeting your minimum daily exercise requirement; the other is that you may have to shop and cook more than you're used to. Although both of these commitments take time, there is no better way to spend your time than doing what needs to be done to take care of your health.

The all-out approach means putting yourself first, which may be hard for people who take care of everyone else's needs before their own. But here's the deal: The food you will be preparing tastes good and it's good for everyone, so if your family or roommates want to join in, fine. If they want to stick with their old routine, this is also fine; but this is what you're cooking for dinner. The all-out approach isn't easy, but the important things in life are worth working for. I will give you as much help as I can with adapting the plan to fit into your own life. But, again, your own dietitian or diabetes educator is the best helper you can get right now.

DASHING TO A MEDITERRANEAN-STYLE DIET

So you want to adapt your present diet to the recommendations in this book without following the meal plans to the letter? Suppose you already count calories, and 1,500 calories a day works for you. The 30 percent of calories that would come from fat on a Mediterranean-style diet is 450 calories, or a fat allowance of 50 grams (450 calories divided by 9 calories per gram of fat).

Since you would use no more than 4 ounces of very lean meat, chicken, or pork containing 2 to 3 grams of fat an ounce, this would use about 8 to 10 grams of fat, leaving about 40 grams to spend on monounsaturated and omega-3s, the good fats. The good fat choices listed below each contain 5 grams of fat for the amounts given, so during the day, you could select eight choices.

GOOD FAT CHOICES

Each choice contains 5 grams of fat and 45 calories

Flaxseed, ground	2 teaspoons
Nuts: pecans or walnuts	4 halves
almonds, cashews, or pistachios	6 nuts
Oil (olive, canola, flaxseed, nut oils)	1 teaspoon
Olives, green stuffed	10 large olives

Olives, large black	8 large olives
Peanut butter	2 teaspoons
Peanuts	10 nuts
Sesame seeds	1 tablespoon

Note: If your weight, LDL and total cholesterol, blood glucose, and triglyceride values are all very high, and your HDL cholesterol is low, it may even be advisable to increase the percentage of calories from fat beyond 30 percent. But in this case you need the help of your own registered dietitian because this strategy works only if the good fats are replacing refined carbohydrates in your diet.

In addition to the good fats, the eating pattern is similar to the DASH diet (page 84), which includes 2 to 3 servings of low-fat dairy products and 8 to 10 servings of fruits and vegetables a day. My advice is to concentrate on vegetables; they are lower in carbohydrates and therefore lower in calories than fruits, not to mention all their wonderful phytochemicals and fiber. And you can now buy carrots and other packaged vegetables ready to eat so you can actually say fresh and convenient in the same sentence. To round out your eating plan, the other emphasis should be on eating high-fiber whole grains and beans.

—ROBIN EDELMAN,
Registered Dietitian, Certified Diabetes Educator, and Vegetable Enthusiast

STOCKING THE HEALTHY PANTRY

Meals do not always have to be difficult to prepare or exclusively fresh off the vine to be good for you. Sure, it would be nice if we could all step out the door and pick organic vegetables and catch a couple of fresh trout for dinner, but this simply is not realistic. What we do have is an incredible abundance of foods available to us—preserved and fresh—including everything you need to eat like a Mediterranean. Keeping these foods on hand and learning what to do with them are the final steps. Here, I'll take you through the supermarket and describe all the foods you will need, how to use them, why they're good for you, and how many of them are great time savers

Artichoke Hearts

I have to admit, I've never prepared fresh artichokes at home because I don't find whole artichokes tasty enough to go to all that expense and work. But canned artichokes hearts are another story. To me, the hearts are the best part, and all the work is already done; so all you need to do is open the can, drain, and rinse them. And ½ cup of canned artichokes has only about 40 calories and no fat. They are great in salads; on pizza; and in pasta dishes, such as Shrimp and Artichokes with Lemony Pasta (page 179). Look for artichokes packed in water, not in oil, because the reasonably priced brand of marinated artichokes contains hydrogenated oils. If you want to make your own, check out the recipe for Artichoke Hearts and Carmelized Onions (page 145).

Balsamic Vinegar

Balsamic vinegar, a rich, dark brown wine vinegar, originated in northern Italy and was once aged in oak barrels for at least ten, and sometimes as long as a hundred years. Because balsamic vinegar is less acidic and sweeter than other vinegars, less oil is needed in salad dressings to balance its acidity. Really great imported balsamic vinegar is very expensive, but there are many less expensive brands that are also very good. We use so much balsamic vinegar that I use one part apple cider vinegar to one part balsamic vinegar in salad dressings to cut down on the expense.

Bread

All or most of the bread you eat should be made from whole grains, one of the prime sources of fiber and trace minerals in our diet. Breads baked with white or refined flour are nutritionally inferior because they are made from what is left after the fiber and most of the nutrients have been stripped from the wheat. And don't forget how much more full and satisfied you feel after eating a sandwich made with whole wheat, compared to a sandwich made with white bread.

The tricky part about selecting a good bread is that you can't tell from the nutrition facts on the label which breads are made from whole wheat and which are made from refined wheat. But there's a foolproof way to find out: Check the ingredient list. Because ingredients are listed in descending order by amount, the first ingredient should be "whole wheat flour." If you see "wheat flour" listed first, don't be fooled; this means that the bread is made from mostly white flour because white flour *is* wheat flour. (Sometimes breads made with white flour have caramel added to make them look brown.) White flour may also be referred to as "unbleached" or "enriched." The key word to look for is "whole"; the real thing may also be called "100% whole wheat flour" or "stone-ground whole wheat flour."

Oats and rye are two other whole-grain ingredients to look for. Whereas wheat is high in insoluble fiber, the type of fiber that keeps you regular and helps fill you up, oats and rye are high in soluble fiber, the type that slows the rise in blood glucose after a meal. Ideal breads contain whole wheat and oats, whole wheat and rye, or even all three. Keep in mind, however, that whole wheat flour will usually appear first in the ingredient list because bread needs a protein in wheat (gluten) to rise properly. Oats and rye are too low in gluten to make bread rise on their own.

Canned Beans

A variety of plain canned beans is essential to the healthy pantry; not only are many more types of canned beans available than dried, but they are available perfectly cooked with just a spin of the can opener. If you've ever faithfully followed the long, drawn-out cooking process for preparing dried beans only to have them come out mushy or as hard, tasteless pellets, you know what a convenience canned beans can be. Besides, there's no reason to have health qualms about making the switch—canned beans have the same nutritional advantages as homemade:

- **High in soluble fiber.** Beans are among the richest source of soluble fiber, the kind that helps temper your blood sugar levels after a meal. Most canned beans contain 7 to 8 grams of fiber per cup.

- **A source of plant proteins.** Beans have been a source of inexpensive plant protein, "poor man's meat," since ancient times. Today it is known that eating more plant protein and less animal protein helps fight chronic diseases.

- **Fat profile: excellent.** Whether home cooked or canned, pinto beans, soldier beans, black beans, lima beans, kidney beans, great Northern beans, and chickpeas (garbanzo beans) all contain 1 gram of fat or less, and about 0.2 gram of saturated fat.

Note: Always rinse canned beans before adding them to a recipe. The cloudy liquid contains added salt and indigestible sugars that cause intestinal gas. The recipes in this book call for red kidney beans, great Northern beans, black beans, or chickpeas.

Canola Oil

There is really no trick to buying canola oil, except to buy it in small quantities so you don't get stuck with a big bottle of two-year-old oil. Canola oil is usually sold in clear containers, so make sure you store it in a cool, dark cupboard or transfer it to a lightproof oil tin. This goes for any oil sold in a clear container, because light and heat speed up the oxidation process and makes fats go rancid quicker.

Canola Oil Spread

Regular margarine contains varying amounts of hydrogenated oils (and trans fats), but there is at least one spread completely free of hydrogenated oils that is made from canola oil thickened with soluble fibers (xanthan and guar gums). The brand name is Spectrum Naturals; and although it was once found only in health food stores, it is now turning up at supermarkets across the country. This means that consumer demand for products free of hydrogenated oils is on the rise, and also suggests that there may soon be other brands available.

Chicken Broth

Because many recipes call for less than a can of chicken broth, those new 32-ounce reclosable cartons of chicken broth are a beautiful thing. You open a carton, use what you need, and pop the rest into the refrigerator where it will be whenever you need more. The broth is already defatted, so you don't have to worry about skimming off the fat; and reduced-sodium broth is also available. If you need to restrict sodium, however, keep in mind that even reduced-sodium chicken broth is quite high in salt, so use it sparingly or make your own. Freeze homemade chicken broth—or leftover canned broth you won't use within two weeks—in ice cube trays, which is another good way to have just what you need on hand.

Chipotle Peppers

Canned chipotle peppers, which are jalapeño peppers that have been dried and smoked, can usually be found in the Mexican food section of the supermarket. With their smoky, hot, sweet, almost chocolaty flavor, canned chipotles in adobo sauce are a great addition to recipes that call for a little heat. Remove the seeds to keep the heat down, chop them finely, and add chipotles to chili and other bean dishes along with a bit of the adobo sauce. You will probably use only one or two chipotles at a time, so store the leftovers in a glass jar in the refrigerator, where they will keep for over a month.

Crackers

Crackers free of hydrogenated oils are not that easy to find except in health food stores, but there are at least two types available in supermarkets. One type is a crisp bread, sold under the brand names Wasa and Ry-Krisp, that is high in fiber and has no added fat. The other is a line of snack crackers from Frookie made with organic whole wheat flour and liquid (not hydrogenated) oils. You may find other crackers made with whole grains and good oils; check the ingredient list to find out, and check the nutrition facts for the calorie and fiber count. For the meal plans in Chapter 12, I used Wasa rye crackers, which have just 45 calories and 3 grams of fiber in two crackers. (If you can find them, the ones with sun-dried tomatoes are really good.) Graham crackers and gingersnaps from Mi-Del are also free of hydrogenated oils; however, because supermarket brands of these snacks are low in total fat, they are also low in trans fats, so if you eat the more common brands once in a while, it's not the end of the world.

Flaxseeds

Flaxseeds have been consumed for centuries in the Mediterranean and other parts of Europe, but they have been virtually unknown in this country until quite recently, except among the health food crowd, where they have long been known as a natural laxative. Flaxseeds have become more well known lately because they have cancer-fighting properties, contain phytochemicals called lignans, and are the most concentrated plant source of omega-3 fatty acids. You can buy these pleasant-tasting nutty little seeds in the health food section of your supermarket or at the health food store; and like nuts, they keep best if stored in the freezer. (Note: Don't eat more than 3 tablespoons of flaxseeds a day. They contain a substance that interferes with the body's use of iodine.) Toasted, flaxseeds can be added to baked goods or sprinkled on cereal. You can also get your flaxseed fix from Uncle Sam cereal (made by U.S. Mills in Omaha, Nebraska), which also happens to be a great whole-grain cereal. And because flaxseeds are fast growing in popularity, you may be able to find good whole-grain bread with the flaxseeds baked right in.

Flaxseed Oil

Flaxseed oil is even more concentrated in omega-3s than are the seeds, and it is becoming a popular addition to healthy shakes and smoothies. Flaxseed oil, however, does not keep very well because it is high in polyunsaturated fat, so it is always better to buy it in small amounts and store it in the refrigerator. If you decide to supplement your diet with flaxseed oil on a regular basis, keep in mind that it is pure fat, so like other oils, it contains about 45 calories a teaspoon.

Frozen Greens

There's nothing like fresh greens for a salad, but when it comes to soups, casseroles, and even spinach pie, frozen can't be beat. It takes many cups of fresh spinach to make a 1-pound bag of frozen spinach. And with frozen spinach, you don't have to stand over the sink, picking off the stems and icky leaves, only to watch what's left shrink to nothing after it's cooked. Look for frozen spinach in a bag, because you can take out just as much as you need to pop into the soup, and put the rest back in the freezer. And although frozen spinach is definitely a staple, you can often find frozen collard, mustard, and beet greens. Substitute these greens for frozen spinach in recipes or add them straight from the freezer into soups. There's no easier way to get a boost of disease-fighting phytochemicals.

Fruit Preserves

Fruit preserves are widely available in all-fruit and reduced-sugar versions. A very good brand of reduced-sugar preserves that is widely available is Smucker's, which seems to have more fruit than other brands, particularly in the strawberry preserves. And although it contains half the carbohydrates of regular preserves (6 versus 12 grams), it tastes just as sweet. Although sugar is okay in reasonable amounts, I think this product is worth buying if you include fruit preserves in your diet on a regular basis. If you add some strawberry preserves to plain nonfat yogurt, the result tastes better and is lower in calories than the presweetened fruit yogurts. I also use this brand of preserves in the topping for Strawberry Cheese Pie (page 209).

Garlic

No one really knows how much of the good health enjoyed by Mediterraneans comes from their love of garlic, but scientists who study the medicinal value of plants usually place garlic number one in the phytochemical hit parade. And equal to garlic's health benefits is its taste. Roasted in a hot oven, garlic becomes sweet, mellow, and almost buttery. In fact, you can do your heart a favor by spreading it on bread in place of butter. A clove of roasted garlic squeezed into homemade salad dressing adds depth and flavor without the unpleasant bite that can come from raw garlic. Roasted garlic transforms plain mashed potatoes or twice-baked potatoes into something truly special. Once you've tasted roasted garlic, you will probably want to make it a regular habit. See page 136 to learn how.

Hummus

Most brands of store-bought hummus, which you can usually find near the dairy section of your supermarket, are every bit as good as homemade. This creamy, incredibly healthy spread from the Middle Eastern part of the Mediterranean is made from chickpeas, garlic, and tahini (a paste made from sesame seeds). Keep hummus in your refrigerator for quick sandwiches or as a dip with Pita Crisps (page 193). In fact, hummus in a whole-wheat pita pocket, plain or with lettuce and tomato, is one of the healthiest sandwiches you can eat (at our house it's second only to p.b. and j.'s). And if you get bored with plain hummus, you can find interesting varieties with added lemon, roasted red peppers, olives, roasted garlic, or cracked black pepper. If you go through as much hummus as we do, it's worth it to make your own. See page 189 for my easy recipe that uses peanut butter instead of tahini.

Italian Turkey Sausage

Both sweet and hot Italian turkey sausages are available in most supermarkets, either refrigerated in the meat section or in the frozen food case. Even though turkey sausage has a fraction of the saturated fat of regular sausage, it adds great flavor to casseroles, sauces, and soups from its Italian seasonings. I keep it in the freezer and use it for recipes such as Beans and Greens Casserole (page 163) and Vegetable Lasagna with a Bit of Sausage (page 167).

Nuts

When a heart patient tells me her doctor told her not to eat nuts because they have fat in them, I wonder how long it's been since that doctor opened a medical journal. Nuts are from plants. Nuts contain good monounsaturated fats. Nuts have the full range of nutrients a baby plant needs to start life. Nuts are good. There are even clinical studies showing that adding walnuts, peanuts, and almonds to the diet lowers bad cholesterol and triglycerides without making people gain weight. And keep in mind that walnuts, a favorite in Mediterranean cooking, also contain omega-3 fatty acids (page 64). Buy nuts in bulk to save money; and if you can, taste them to make sure they're fresh. Nuts do get stale, but storing them in the freezer keeps them fresh. In fact, it is a good idea to weigh out 1-ounce parcels of nuts and freeze them so you can grab them in the morning to take with you for snacks. Yes, nuts are the ideal snack. Even though they are calorie dense, there are few things more satisfying and good for your blood sugar and cholesterol. Pop Quiz: What do you think is better for you between meals when you are really hungry? Cookies from the vending machine or a handful of nuts?

Oat Bran Cereal

Oat bran is the part of the oat that contains the most soluble fiber, so using it in recipes such as Breakfast Cakes (page 187) helps make them as effective as they can be at lowering blood glucose and cholesterol. Oat bran cereal can also be eaten as a hot cereal.

Oatmeal

Oats grow too far north to be part of a traditional Mediterranean diet; but because they are rich in soluble fiber, they certainly are a great addition to our American version of the diet. I use oats in baking and as the main grain in my baked goods and dessert recipes to boost the soluble fiber, which helps temper the rise in blood glucose. Most of my recipes call for quick-cooking oats, which are simply old-fashioned oats that have been cut smaller than normal so they cook more quickly; and I find that they work well for baking. (Please note that quick-cooking oats are *not* the same as instant oats, which cannot be used as a substitute because they have been precooked.) Old-fashioned oatmeal can usually replace quick-cooking oatmeal in recipes; however, I usually buy large containers of quick-cooking rolled oats, which can be used in all of the recipes.

Olive Oil

About five years ago, I went through my cupboards and threw out all the oils and replaced them with a gallon tin of light olive oil. I suggest you do the same. (If you haven't read Chapters 5 and 8, that's where to go to find out why.) Since then, I also began buying canola oil for baking and extra-virgin olive oil for special recipes. Light olive oil is not lower in fat than other olive oils, and it is lighter in color because the tiny bits of solids from the original olives have been removed. Extra-virgin olive oil (sometimes referred to as cold-pressed) is from the first pressing of the olives, which gives it the wonderful flavor and color of olives. These very fine oils are expensive, because they don't retain their full flavor longer than a few months after harvest; but if you know how to choose them they are certainly worth it. I'm no expert, but I do know that it's best to store all oil in dark bottles or light-proof containers, which helps protect them from oxidation. Use good olive oil when the flavor will be noticeable, on special salads or on bread, and light olive oil for everyday cooking.

Peanut Butter

Oh, sure, you gave up peanut butter a long time ago because it's high in fat. But like the peanuts it's made from, this versatile legume is perhaps America's greatest contribution to a healthy Mediterranean-style diet. But you don't have to just take my word for it: New research finds that eating peanut products does not make people gain weight—they eat about the same amount of calories as when they are on a peanut-free diet. But their blood fats behave much better with the peanuts than without (page 39). And peanut butter is the ultimate convenience food—it's good for you, it's portable, it's versatile, and kids like it. There's only one shopping tip: Buy peanut butter that is not hydrogenated. You will have to look closely because supermarket brands of unhydrogenated and hydrogenated peanut butter look so much alike. The unhydrogenated product is usually called "natural" or "old-fashioned"; and other than that, the packaging looks identical to the hydrogenated stuff. (If in doubt, check the ingredient list.) To me, the best-tasting peanut butter is made with roasted peanuts, but the best bargains are the supermarket brands, which still taste pretty darn good.

Powdered Egg Whites

Powdered egg whites are great to have on hand for shakes and other recipes that call for uncooked egg whites. Because of the risk of salmonella, it is unsafe to use uncooked raw eggs or egg whites in recipes. Products such as Just Whites, made from pasteurized egg whites, are available in most supermarkets. One can of Just Whites is the equivalent of 4¾ egg whites, and the cost is approximately what you would pay for the same number of fresh eggs.

Prosciutto

The Italian word for "ham," *prosciutto* usually refers to dense, thinly sliced ham that has been seasoned, salt-cured, and air-dried. You can often find prosciutto at the supermarket deli, and most definitely in Italian markets. Recipes that call for prosciutto also work with thinly sliced lean ham; but if you come across the real thing, it is one of those ingredients worth buying once in a while for its wonderful flavor. Yes it is salty, but not terribly fatty and you need only a small amount.

Roasted Red Peppers in a Jar

Like frozen spinach, jarred roasted red peppers are a convenience food you can really love. If you've ever roasted peppers yourself and had to deal with all that black char that sticks to everything, you know what I mean. Besides, fresh red peppers are sometimes so expensive that, pepper for pepper, the jarred kind costs less. And here's the best part: ½ cup of roasted red peppers contains only 25 calories. If you serve them to friends, they'll think you slaved over the meal, and you don't have to tell them the peppers came from a jar.

Sun-Dried Tomatoes

As you might guess, sun-dried tomatoes are dehydrated tomatoes, dried either in the sun the old-fashioned way, or by slowly drying in a low oven. In Italy, small tomatoes are sometimes dried still clinging to the vine by hanging the entire plant to dry in a sunny place. (If you grow tomatoes, you can get seeds for special drying tomatoes by mail order.) Drying tomatoes makes them intensely sweet and flavorful, and they add a wonderful richness to stews and soups. Buy the kind that are sold dry in cellophane, not packed in oil: They are usually less expensive, and if you're going to add oil to your recipe, you should use your own good oil. If the tomatoes are very hard and dry, just soak them in water for a few minutes before using. The easiest way to cut them is to snip them into tiny strips with scissors.

Yogurt

Yogurt is fermented milk. The nice bacteria that turn milk into yogurt, such as *Lactobacillus acidophilus,* are also friendly to your gastrointestinal (GI) tract, so people often eat yogurt to help keep the bad bacteria in check. There is also some evidence that eating yogurt on a regular basis can boost the immune system. At any rate, low-fat and nonfat yogurt are great ingredients for healthy cooking, because they can replace ingredients high in saturated fat (such as sour cream and cream cheese) while providing substantial amounts of calcium and other nutrients. Interestingly, many brands of reduced-fat yogurts have up to 33 percent more calcium than the milk from which they are made (400 versus 300 milligrams per cup) because nonfat milk solids are often added to them as a thickener. When shopping for yogurt to make Yogurt Cheese (page 196), look for the best, sweetest-tasting plain nonfat yogurt you can find. Check the label: Yogurts made with *L. thermophilus* or *L. bulgaricus* and other exotically named cultures are usually relatively sweet; yogurts made with *L. acidophilus* alone tend to be a little tart. (If you can buy Stoneyfield Farm plain yogurt where you live, try it—it's so good you can eat it right out of the carton.) Often, the best yogurt comes from your local organic dairy. One more thing to check: The label should say "made with live yogurt cultures"; if it has been heat-treated, the beneficial bacteria are dead and they can do you no good.

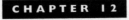

CHAPTER 12

♥

The Meal Plans

Following someone else's meal plans to the letter is not necessary for a healthy diet; in fact, the best plan is one you create yourself. But you have to start somewhere, and this fourteen-day Mediterranean-style eating pattern is designed to show you how to bring all of the nutrition pieces together.

The plan takes into account the nutrition research described in the first ten chapters, particularly the Seven Countries Study, the Lyon Diet Heart Study, the fiber studies, the DASH diet study, and the research on heart disease and insulin resistance. But, as they say, the proof is in the pudding; after six weeks you will see for yourself how the Good Fat Diet affects what really matters: your weight, blood sugar, cholesterol, and triglycerides and, not in the least, how you feel.

THE COMPOSITION OF THE DIET

In a nutshell, the diet is a 1,500-calorie plan with an ideal balance of protein, good fats, carbohydrates, and fiber. The fat content averages around 30 percent of calories, which is higher than many so-called low-fat diets, in which calories from fat can be as low as 10 percent. Of course, what happens when you keep the proportion of fat that low is that the proportion of carbohydrates is necessarily higher, generally falling between 70 and 75 percent, which, as we have seen, is not a good idea for people battling high blood sugar and/or high triglycerides. On the other hand, the Good Fat Diet is not a high-fat diet (30 percent of calories is the upper limit of most health recommendations). A true Mediterranean diet could actually be higher in good fats and still be healthy, if calories were not an issue. But when calories are limited, a little less fat translates to a greater volume of food, so keeping the fat to the 30 percent level makes those calories go farther. Here's how the average calories in the plan break down:

Protein:	**20%**
Fats:	**30% (saturated < 7%)**
Carbohydrates:	**50%**

For blood pressure control, the plan is also as high in calcium, potassium, and magnesium as possible, while sodium easily falls below the recommended limit of 2,400 milligrams a day:

Calcium:	**1,100 milligrams**
Potassium:	**3,600 milligrams**
Magnesium:	**390 milligrams**

And last but not least, the dietary fiber content of the plan averages 25 grams a day, which is quite high for a 1,500-calorie diet, when you consider that the average American eats many more calories and yet takes in only about 11 grams of fiber a day.

GETTING STARTED

This section is for people who are taking the all-out approach of following the meal plans for six weeks. In effect, you will be running a diet study, in which you will be the sole subject. (If you're just starting out with your walking plan, you will be running a diet and exercise study.)

Plan a visit to your doctor ahead of time, and also plan to spend a good part of a weekend to get your first set of goals down on paper, to shop, and to prepare some make-ahead recipes. Don't worry, it will be easier the second week; and before long, you will know your pattern so well you that you'll be able to whip up a shopping list in no time. But in the beginning, you really need time to learn about new foods and to think about the combinations that will work for you. You'll also probably need to spend a few hours in the supermarket looking for new products and reading labels. Your health is worth it.

Step 1

Explain to your doctor what you want to do, and ask him or her to do the relevant tests before you start: blood cholesterol profile, blood pressure, triglycerides, fasting glucose, and Hemoglobin Alc (HbAlc), a test that shows how well your blood sugar is controlled over time. You will need the results to see how well the diet works. Discuss the supplements recommended in the diet plan (Chapter 9) to see if there are any reasons that they shouldn't be recommended for you. When your doctor gives the okay, you don't have to wait for the test results, you can go on to the next step.

Step 2

Review the meal plans carefully and the recipes that go with them, choosing seven plans that contain foods and food combinations that sound appealing to you. Then check the recipes that go with the plans (the page numbers for the recipes are given in parentheses) and make sure these are dishes you want to try. Next, if you haven't already been keeping a log, set up a notebook to keep track of your daily exercise; daily food intake; weekly weight; and if needed, your blood glucose record. When you receive the test report from your doctor, record the numbers on a separate page in your notebook. Keeping good records is how you will track all your hard work and the results of your efforts.

Go over the meal plans you have chosen. If there are any meals or snacks that you're really not crazy about, refer to "Mix-and-Match Meals" (page 125) to find an alternative for that particular item. The system is set up so that the replacement meals and snacks will not be higher in calories than those in the main plan, but they might be a little lower. When you come up with a seven-day plan that sounds good, you are ready to make a shopping list. Read over "Questions and Answers" (page 213) to get a good understanding of why certain foods and recipes have been chosen for the meal plans.

Step 3

After you have a seven-day plan you like, you can go ahead and make your shopping list, but make sure you have read "Stocking the Healthy Pantry" (page 96) so you know what products to look for. (If you have specific questions that are not addressed in Chapter 11 and do not have a dietitian available, call the American Dietetic Association nutrition hotline at 900-225-5267, where you can get your questions answered for a small fee.) Most of the recipes make four servings, so if you are cooking for one, you will probably want to cut them in half, and have the leftovers the next day or freeze them for future use. If you have a full-time, five-day workweek, it would be ideal if for the first time around, you did your planning and shopping on Saturday and prepared your make-ahead food on Sunday to get ready for the week ahead. One last thing before you begin: Be flexible. Life sometimes gets in the way, so if something doesn't work out, use your knowledge of nutrition to make other good choices; if you have a bad day, see what you can do to make the next one better. As I've said over and over, there's nothing magical about this plan—the magic comes from you and your determination to eat for your health. It will be hard work in the beginning, but it will get easier.

RECOMMENDED SUPPLEMENTS

❂ *Multi-vitamin-mineral supplement*

❂ *200 to 250 milligrams vitamin C*

❂ *100 to 400 milligrams vitamin E*

❂ *Calcium as needed*

❂ *Make sure your physician approves all supplements other than th multivitamin.*

For more specific information on choosing supplements, see Chapter 9

Beverages

Yes!! Get the recommended eight glasses of water (fluid) a day. This is particularly important if you are going from a low-fiber diet to a high-fiber diet. Other than skim milk, all beverages should be noncaloric, unless you make the decision to add wine to your plan (page 87). Good choices are given in the "Free Food and Beverage List."

FREE FOOD AND BEVERAGE LIST

The following foods and beverages can be added to your meal plans at your discretion:

Coffee

Cereal-based hot beverages (e.g., Postum, Cafex)

Diet soda

Dill pickles (limit if you are on a sodium restriction)

Garlic

Herbal teas

Herbs

Horseradish

Hot sauce

Ketchup (1 tablespoon)

Lemon

Lemon juice

Lime

Lime juice

Mineral water

Mustard

Noncaloric sweeteners

Sparkling water

Spices

Tea

Vinegar

Wine used in cooking

THE MEAL PLANS

Day 1

Breakfast

1 cup cooked oatmeal

1 tablespoon chopped walnuts

1 teaspoon firmly packed brown sugar

Ground cinnamon to taste

½ cup skim milk

Snack

1 orange

Lunch

TUNA SALAD SANDWICH

2 ounces white albacore tuna mixed with

2 tablespoons reduced-fat mayonnaise

½ fresh tomato, sliced

Optional: onions, lettuce, and/or chopped celery

2 slices whole wheat or whole-grain rye bread

1 cup skim milk

Snack

1 ounce peanuts

Supper

1 serving Chicken Parmesan (page 179)

1 serving Vegetable Antipasto (page 143)

1 slice Easy Garlic Bread (page 193)

1 pear

Day 2

Breakfast

1 serving Peach Almond Smoothie (page 188)

Snack

1 ounce pecans

Lunch

1 serving Vegetable Antipasto (page 143)

1 ounce reduced-fat Cheddar cheese

1 (6-inch) whole wheat pita bread

Snack

¾ cup (6-ounce container) vanilla low-fat yogurt

1 cup berries (strawberries, blueberries and/or raspberries, fresh or frozen)

Supper

1 serving Frittata (page 170)

2 cups mixed greens (page 131)

2 teaspoons Basic Dressing (page 132)

1 cup skim milk

1 serving Pears Baked in Madeira (page 201)

1 serving Yogurt Cream (page 202)

Day 3

Breakfast

1 egg, scrambled or fried in

½ teaspoon olive oil

1 sliced whole wheat toast with

1 teaspoon canola oil spread

1 cup skim milk

Snack

1 orange

Lunch

TURKEY SANDWICH

2 slices whole wheat bread

2 ounces sliced turkey breast

1 tablespoon reduced-fat mayonnaise

½ fresh tomato, sliced

Lettuce

1 cup skim milk

Snack

2 tablespoons Yogurt Cheese Spread (page 196)

2 rye crackers

Supper

1 serving Med-Mex Casserole (page 149)

2 cups fresh spinach

2 teaspoons Basic Dressing (page 132)

1 serving Baked Apples with Crunchy Topping (page 203)

¼ cup (1 serving) Yogurt Cream (page 202)

Day 4

Breakfast

1 Breakfast Cake (page 187)

1 cup skim milk

Snack

I apple

Lunch

I Mediterranean Pocket (page 194)

I cup skim milk

I pear

I ounce low-fat Cheddar cheese

Snack

I ounce peanuts

Supper

I serving Eggplant Parmesan (page 150)

I slice Easy Garlic Bread (page 193)

2 cups mixed greens (page 131)

2 teaspoons Basic Dressing (page 132)

I orange

Day 5

Breakfast

I cup cooked oatmeal

I tablespoon chopped walnuts

I teaspoon firmly packed brown sugar

Ground cinnamon to taste

½ cup skim milk

Snack

I orange

Lunch

CHICKEN SALAD SANDWICH

2 ounces cooked cubed chicken mixed with

2 tablespoons reduced-fat mayonnaise

Lettuce

2 slices whole wheat bread

I cup skim milk

Snack

I ounce peanuts

Supper

I serving of The Big Salad (page 130)

I serving Red Lentil and Rice Soup (page 171)

2 rye crackers

Day 6

Breakfast

I slice whole wheat toast

I tablespoon peanut butter

I teaspoon fruit preserves

I cup skim milk

Snack

I orange

Lunch

2 rye crackers

2 ounces reduced-fat Cheddar cheese

I serving Red Lentil and Rice Soup (page 171)

I apple

Snack

6 baby carrots

2 tablespoons Yogurt-Mustard Dip (page 191)

Supper

1 serving Spinach Pie (page 152)

1 serving Summer Tomato Salad (page 134)

1 slice whole-grain rye bread with

1 teaspoon canola oil spread

½ cup sliced peaches, fresh or canned in light syrup with

¼ cup (1 serving) Yogurt Cream (page 202)

Day 7

Breakfast

1 serving Peach Almond Smoothie (page 188)

Snack

1 rice, corn, or wheat cake

2 teaspoons peanut butter

Lunch

1 serving Spinach Pie (page 152)

1 cup skim milk

1 apple

Snack

1 ounce pistachio nuts

Supper

1 serving Chicken Cassoulet (page 176)

1 cup steamed whole green beans, fresh or frozen

1 slice whole wheat bread

1 teaspoon canola oil spread

1 serving Crunchy Baked Bananas (page 212)

Day 8

Breakfast

1 cup cooked oatmeal

1 teaspoon firmly packed brown sugar

Ground cinnamon to taste

2 tablespoon chopped walnuts

½ cup skim milk

Snack

1 orange

Lunch

AVOCADO AND TOMATO SANDWICH

2 slices whole wheat bread

2 ounces sliced avocado (about one-third of a small avocado)

1 small plum tomato, sliced

Lettuce

1 tablespoon reduced-fat mayonnaise

1 cup skim milk

Snack

6 baby carrots

2 tablespoons Yogurt-Mustard Dip (page 191)

Supper

1 serving Red Beans and Rice (page 166)

2 cups mixed greens (page 131) with

1 ounce crumbled feta cheese

2 tablespoons Basic Dressing (page 132)

1 cup skim milk

2 Pecan Currant Drops (page 207)

Day 9

Breakfast

1 slice whole wheat toast

1 tablespoon peanut butter

1 cup skim milk

1 orange

Snack

1 ounce pecans

Lunch

TURKEY SANDWICH

2 slices whole wheat bread

2 ounces sliced turkey breast

1 tablespoon reduced-fat mayonnaise

½ fresh tomato, sliced

Lettuce

1 cup skim milk

1 banana

Snack

1 serving Chivey Cheese Spread (page 198)

2 rye crackers

Supper

1 serving Lentils and Bulgur with Walnuts (page 157)

1 serving Oven-Braised Carrots and Green Onions (page 141)

I cup skim milk

2 Chocolate Hazelnut Drops (page 208)

Day 10

Breakfast
I slice whole wheat toast

I tablespoon peanut butter

I cup skim milk

Snack
I orange

Lunch

HUMMUS SANDWICH

¼ cup hummus, store bought or homemade (page 189)

2 slices whole wheat bread

½ tomato, sliced

I apple

Lettuce

I cup skim milk

Snack
¼ cup dry roasted mixed nuts

Supper
I serving Mediterranean Fish Bake (page 183)

I slice Easy Garlic Bread (page 193)

I serving Spinach Salad (page 138)

I cup skim milk

I pear

Day 11

Breakfast

1 egg scrambled or fried in

1 teaspoon olive oil

1 ounce Canadian bacon

1 slice whole wheat toast

1 cup skim milk

Snack

1 banana

Lunch

1 serving Black Beans and Rice Salad (page 140)

1 ounce sliced avocado (about one-third of a small avocado)

4 whole-grain crackers

1 apple

Snack

1 cup skim milk

2 graham crackers

1 tablespoon peanut butter

Supper

1 serving Turkey Marsala (page 177)

1 slice Easy Garlic Bread (page 193)

1 serving Spinach Salad (page 138)

1 serving Oven-Braised Carrots and Green Onions (page 141)

1 cup skim milk

Day 12

Breakfast

1 serving Peach Almond Smoothie (page 188)

Snack

1 ounce pistachio nuts

Lunch

AVOCADO AND TOMATO SANDWICH

2 slices whole wheat bread

2 ounces sliced avocado (about one-third of a small avocado)

1 small plum tomato, sliced

Lettuce

1 tablespoon reduced-fat mayonnaise

1 cup skim milk

1 pear

Snack

4 tablespoons Yogurt Cheese Spread (page 202)

4 rye crackers

Supper

3 ounces baked or roasted chicken breast, no skin

1 serving Lemony Roasted Asparagus (page 142)

1 serving Roasted Potato Sticks (page 137)

1 orange

Day 13

Breakfast

1 cup cooked oatmeal

1 tablespoon chopped walnuts

1 teaspoon firmly packed brown sugar

Ground cinnamon to taste

½ cup skim milk

Snack

1 ounce roasted peanuts

1 apple

Lunch

HUMMUS SANDWICH

¼ cup hummus, store bought or homemade (page 189)

2 slices whole wheat bread

½ tomato, sliced

Lettuce

1 hard-boiled egg

1 cup skim milk

Snack

1 ounce reduced-fat Cheddar cheese

2 rye crackers

Supper

1 serving Simple Salmon (page 181)

1 cup steamed whole green beans, fresh or frozen

1 serving Winter Slaw (page 133)

I slice whole-grain rye bread with

I teaspoon canola oil spread

I cup strawberries with

½ cup (2 servings) Yogurt Cream (page 202)

Day 14

Breakfast

I slice whole wheat toast

I tablespoon peanut butter

I cup skim milk

Snack

I orange

Lunch

I serving Mediterranean Tuna Salad (page 184)

I rye cracker

I pear

Snack

I cup skim milk

I rice, corn, or wheat cake

2 teaspoons almond or peanut butter

Supper

I serving Chicken Cacciatore (page 175)

2 slices Easy Garlic Bread (page 193)

2 cups mixed greens (page 131)

2 teaspoons Basic Dressing (page 132)

I apple

HOW TO CUSTOMIZE YOUR MEAL PLAN

1. If you prefer not to have snacks, simply include the snack items with the meals.

2. If the fruit listed is not available, substitute another piece of fresh fruit. Do not substitute fruit juice for fresh fruit—you need the fiber to help with weight loss, lowering blood sugar, lowering blood cholesterol, and keeping the muscle tone in your GI tract in top form. Canned or frozen fruit is an acceptable option. One serving of fruit should have 60 to 80 calories.

3. Instead of preparing a recipe for a vegetable dish or a fruit dessert that appears on the meal plan, when you're short on time, you can substitute a simpler version that contains the same ingredients. For example, for Lemony Roasted Asparagus, it is okay to substitute plain roasted asparagus or even steamed asparagus (starting with fresh or frozen) and adding the same amount of olive oil. In fact, if you hate asparagus, you could substitute another vegetable, such as green beans, which has a similar nutritional profile. Another example is Pears Baked in Madeira; here you could just have a half of a pear and ½ cup plain nonfat yogurt with a touch of sweetener. The plain versions certainly won't taste as good, but you may not always have preparation time.

4. The other option is substituting meals in the following section for meals in the meal plans. These substitutions are designed to have about the same or fewer calories than the meals they are replacing.

5. **Use common sense:** Armed with your own book of food values, available at any bookstore, you will learn to make your own substitutions. When you do, always consider three things: calories, type of fat, and fiber. Over time, your meal plans will evolve into a pattern that is truly yours, complete with some of your own recipes.

MIX-AND-MATCH MEALS

Breakfasts

Each of the following meals contains around 300 calories.

1. 1 Breakfast Cake (page 187)

   1 cup skim milk or 1 cup nonfat yogurt

2. 1 Peach Almond Smoothie (page 188)

3. 1 (6-inch) whole wheat pita, toasted

   1 ounce part-skim mozzarella cheese

   ½ sliced tomato

   1 orange

   1 cup skim milk or 1 cup nonfat yogurt

4. 1 slice whole wheat toast

   1 tablespoon peanut butter

   1 cup skim milk or 1 cup nonfat yogurt

   1 orange

5. 1 egg or ¼ cup egg substitute cooked in

   1 teaspoon olive oil

   1 (1-ounce) slice Canadian bacon

   2 slices whole wheat toast

Lunches

Each of the following meals contains around 400 calories.

1. 1 cup canned lentil soup

   2 Parmesan Crisps (page 195) or

   3 rye crackers

1 cup skim milk or 1 cup nonfat yogurt

1 pear

2. 1 Mediterranean Pocket (page 194)

   1 cup skim milk or 1 cup nonfat yogurt

   1 ounce cashews

3. 2 ounces white albacore tuna mixed with

   2 tablespoons reduced-fat mayonnaise

   Optional: onions, lettuce, and/or chopped celery

   2 slices whole wheat or whole-grain rye bread

   1 cup skim milk or 1 cup nonfat yogurt

   1 apple

4. ¼ cup hummus, store bought or homemade (page 189)

   2 slices whole wheat bread

   ½ tomato, sliced

   Lettuce

   1 cup skim milk

   ½ banana

5. 2 slices whole wheat bread

   2 ounces sliced turkey breast

   1 tablespoon reduced-fat mayonnaise

   ½ fresh tomato, sliced

   Lettuce

   1 cup skim milk

   2 ounces grapes

Suppers

Each of the following meals contains around 400 calories.

1. 1 serving Simple Salmon (page 181)

   1 serving Mess o' Greens (page 135)

   1 serving Roasted Potato Sticks (page 137)

2. 1 serving Frittata (page 170)

   1 serving Roasted Plum Tomatoes (page 146)

   1 serving Spinach Salad (page 138)

   1 (6-inch) whole wheat pita bread

   1 teaspoon canola oil spread

3. 3 ounces roasted or baked chicken breast, skin removed

   ½ baked potato

   ¼ cup Yogurt Cheese (page 196) with chopped chives, if desired

   1 cup steamed green beans, fresh or frozen

   1 teaspoon canola oil spread

   1 slice whole-grain rye bread

   1 apple

4. 1 serving Mediterranean Fish Bake (page 183)

   2 cups mesclun (page 131), or other greens

   1 ounce sliced avocado (about one-third of a small avocado)

   2 teaspoons Basic Dressing (page 132)

   1 (6-inch) whole wheat pita bread

5. 1 serving Vegetable Pie (page 151)

   1 serving Artichoke Hearts and Caramelized Onions (page 145)

   1 serving Baked Apples with Crunchy Topping (page 203)

   ¼ cup Yogurt Cream (page 202)

CHAPTER 13

♥

Salads and Vegetable Dishes

At one time, my vegetable know-how was limited to steamed broccoli. But around the time I went to work for *Eating Well* magazine, a whole new world opened up for me. Not only did I start seeing report after report about the cancer-fighting substances in different vegetables, I also learned so many great new ways of preparing them that I was able to leave steamed broccoli—which I never really cared for anyway—behind forever.

Instead of being relegated to a side-dish chapter, vegetables star in these first three recipe chapters, because they are the first thing we should think about when planning meals. And it's not just because they are low in calories, high in fiber, and rich in vitamins and minerals. Vegetables contain literally hundreds of phytochemicals (plant chemicals) that protect us against disease. In fact, experts say that eating vegetables and other plant foods is the single most powerful way to protect ourselves against cancer— as powerful as not smoking!

And, of course, people eating plant-based diets also have less type 2 diabetes and heart disease. Do the phytochemicals in vegetables help here too? Although scientists still have a lot to learn, we do know that vegetables contain a variety of antioxidants, which are likely to protect against oxidative damage caused by high blood sugar and high LDL cholesterol. And we do know that a diet rich in plant foods is lower in calories and higher in fiber than a diet of refined processed foods—exactly the type of diet that helps prevent type 2 diabetes, heart disease, and cancer.

THE BIG SALAD

....

If you adopt only one eating habit from this book, please make it eating salad—not iceberg lettuce and rock-hard orange tomatoes with diet dressing, but wonderful-tasting salads of many vegetables with real dressing. With whole-grain bread, the salad given here can be a full meal, not to mention a plateful of fiber, nutrients, and phytochemicals that is tough to match.

> 6 cups greens, such as loose-leaf red lettuce, spinach, or mesclun (page 131)
>
> ½ cup shredded red cabbage
>
> 2 tablespoons chopped walnuts or pecans
>
> 1 red bell pepper, seeded and sliced, or 1 large ripe tomato, sliced
>
> 1 medium carrot, shredded or sliced
>
> 1 small red onion, thinly sliced
>
> 1 (7½-ounce) can chickpeas, drained and rinsed
>
> 2 tablespoons Basic Dressing (page 132)

1. Wash and dry the greens; tear or cut large leaves into bite-sized pieces. Mix with the cabbage in a large salad bowl or platter.

2. Toast the nuts in a dry skillet over medium heat, stirring occasionally until fragrant, about 5 minutes. Cool.

3. Add the pepper, carrot, onion, and chickpeas to the greens. When the nuts have cooled, sprinkle them over the salad. Toss with the Basic Dressing and serve immediately.

MAKES 2 SERVINGS

280 calories per serving, 11 g protein, 13 g fat (1.5 sat), 36 g carbohydrate, 507 mg sodium, 1,205 mg potassium, 11 g dietary fiber

Exchanges: 3 Vegetable, ½ Lean Meat, 2½ Fat

Variations

℧ For a side salad to go with another entrée, decrease the amount of vegetables and leave out the nuts and chickpeas.

℧ Add any fresh vegetable in season (a greater variety improves the nutritional profile and does little to change the calories). I sometimes add fresh cauliflower florets broken into tiny chunks, artichoke hearts, or lightly steamed asparagus.

℧ Red or white kidney beans (or any favorite bean) can stand in for the chickpeas.

MEET MESCLUN

No, it's not a drug—mesclun is just a fancy French name for a mixture of baby greens, which usually includes spinach, beet greens, arugula, and a variety of other edible leafy vegetables. Mesclun can be expensive, depending on the time of year and where you live; but keep in mind, it's sold ready to go, with no waste. So unless it gets up near ten dollars a pound, as it sometimes does in the winter, it's well worth the price because of its gold mine of vitamins (particularly folate), plant omega-3 fatty acids, and other protective phytochemicals. *Mangiafolia*—eat greens as they do in Italy.

BASIC DRESSING

....

Use a glass canning jar marked in 1-ounce increments for measuring the ingredients (1 ounce = 2 tablespoons) and storing the leftovers.

½ cup olive oil

¼ cup balsamic vinegar

¼ cup apple cider vinegar

2 tablespoons coarse-grained mustard

1 tablespoon pure maple syrup or ½ teaspoon sugar

2 teaspoons dried basil

Salt and freshly ground black pepper to taste

Mix all the ingredients in the jar; secure the lid, and shake well. Store leftover dressing in the refrigerator and bring to room temperature before serving.

MAKES 1¼ CUPS

55 calories per tbsp, 0 g protein, 6 g fat (0.7 sat), 2 g carbohydrate, 22 mg sodium 20 mg potassium, 0 g dietary fiber

Exchanges: 1 Fat

Variations

◊ **ROASTED GARLIC DRESSING.** Mash one or two cloves of roasted garlic (page 136) and whisk into the Basic Dressing.

◊ **REDUCED-CALORIE DRESSING.** If you would like to save your fat calories to spend somewhere else, replace ¼ cup of the olive oil with ¼ cup brewed green or black tea. This makes 1¼ cups dressing with 30 calories and 3 grams fat (0.4 saturated) per tbsp (just under 1 Fat Exchange).

◊ **CREAMY DRESSING.** My children like a milder tasting dressing, so I make a creamy batch by adding ¼ cup reduced-fat mayonnaise. This makes 1½ cups dressing with 52 calories and 5 grams of fat (0.6 sat) per tbsp (1 Fat Exchange).

◊ **COMPANY DRESSING.** To keep the cost down, I usually use light olive oil and a one-to-one mixture of apple cider and balsamic vinegars for my Basic

Dressing. For special occasions, I use extra-virgin olive oil and ½ cup balsamic vinegar. (Calories and fat are the same as for the Basic Dressing.)

WINTER SLAW

Summer or winter, a slaw, which is basically a cabbage salad, is a good alternative to green salads. This refreshing slaw is as good on a cold winter night as it is at a summer picnic.

FOR THE DRESSING

1 tablespoon apple cider vinegar

1 tablespoon olive oil

1 tablespoon low-fat mayonnaise

¼ cup canned crushed pineapple

Salt and freshly ground black pepper to taste

FOR THE SLAW

1 large carrot, grated

1 small green or red bell pepper, seeded and thinly sliced

4 cups shredded cabbage

1. Whisk the dressing ingredients together in a small bowl.

2. Place the slaw ingredients in a large bowl, and toss with the dressing until evenly coated. Refrigerated, leftovers keep for about 1 day.

MAKES 4 SERVINGS

80 calories per serving, 2 g protein, 5 g fat (0.5 sat), 10 g carbohydrate, 23 mg sodium, 335 mg potassium, 3 g dietary fiber

Exchanges: 2 Vegetable, I Fat

TIP

If you don't have pineapple, add about ½ teaspoon sugar or equivalent sweetener, or the slaw will be very tart.

SUMMER TOMATO SALAD

The time to eat fresh tomatoes is when they are at their peak; it is also the time to use the best balsamic vinegar and extra-virgin olive oil you can afford.

½ cup loosely packed basil leaves

1 cup loosely packed arugula or other greens

2 tablespoons Company Dressing (page 132)

2 large, juicy tomatoes, preferably from your own garden

Salt and freshly ground black pepper to taste

1. Wash and dry the basil and greens; arrange on a platter. Toss with 1 tablespoon of the Company Dressing.

2. Slice the tomatoes and arrange on the greens. Drizzle the remaining 1 tablespoon of dressing on the tomatoes. Season with salt and pepper.

MAKES 2 SERVINGS

90 calories per serving, 2 g protein, 6 g fat (0.8 sat), 9 g carbohydrate, 40 mg sodium, 440 mg potassium, 3 g dietary fiber

Exchanges: 2 Vegetable, I Fat

Variation

♥ If you would like to turn this salad into a light lunch, top with ¼ cup crumbled feta cheese and 2 slices of crusty whole-grain bread to sop up the dressing. (Total: 200 calories, 6 g protein, 11 g fat (3 sat), 24 g carbohydrate. Exchanges: 2 Vegetable, I Starch, I Medium-Fat Meat, I Fat)

MESS O' GREENS

If you're from the South, you probably know that traditional mess o' greens get their wonderful flavor from bacon fat. Here's a healthier version flavored with lean Canadian bacon and garlic.

1 large bunch beet or collard greens

1 teaspoon olive oil

2 ounces Canadian bacon, finely minced

2 cloves garlic, minced

1. Stem and wash the greens thoroughly, but do not dry (the water clinging to the leaves helps steam them).

2. Heat the oil in a large nonstick skillet. Add the Canadian bacon and cook over medium heat, stirring, for about 2 minutes.

3. Add the greens and garlic and cook, stirring, until the greens are just wilted. Serve immediately.

MAKES 4 SERVINGS

55 calories per serving, 6 g protein, 2 g fat (0.4 sat), 4 g carbohydrate, 250 mg sodium, 684 mg potassium, 3 g dietary fiber

Exchanges: I Vegetable, ½ Lean Meat

ROASTING VEGETABLES

When I was growing up, people ate roasted meat and canned vegetables, which is maybe why we filled up on meat. But what roasting does to meat—producing perfectly cooked, moist food with tasty, crunchy brown bits—it also can do to many vegetables. The high heat of roasting intensifies flavor by caramelizing the sugars on the outside. Nutrients are also preserved rather than lost in cooking water or steam. A few of my favorite types of roasted vegetables appear here and in Chapter 14, but many other vegetables can be roasted by the general technique used in Roasted Carrots and Green Beans (page 138).

ROASTED GARLIC

If you've never tasted roasted garlic, you're in for a treat. It is sweet, mild, and buttery tasting and so low in calories that you will be finding your own creative ways to use it.

    1 head garlic
    1 teaspoon olive oil

1. Preheat oven to 350° F.

2. Rub the entire head of garlic in your hands to loosen and remove the papery outside skin. Slice off the top ¼ inch of the head to expose the tips of the individual cloves.

3. Place the garlic head on a large square of aluminum foil and drizzle the olive oil over the top. Wrap the head tightly, and roast for 45 minutes until the cloves are golden and easily pierced with a fork.

4. When cool, unwrap the garlic, and separate it into cloves. Remove the roasted garlic by squeezing each clove individually.

MAKES 8 TO 10 TEASPOONS

5 calories per teaspoon, 0.2 g protein, 0.2 g fat, 1 g carbohydrate, 1 mg sodium, 12 mg potassium, trace dietary fiber

Exchanges: Free

HOW TO USE ROASTED GARLIC

1. Use as a spread for bread.
2. Make Roasted Garlic Dressing (page 132).
3. Add to mashed potatoes for rave reviews at the Thanksgiving table. (I always roast a head o garlic along with the turkey; at 325° F, it takes about 1 hour.)
4. Add to dips and spreads, such as Roasted Eggplant and Garlic Spread (page 192) and Peanutty Hummus (page 189), for a sweet garlic flavor that even garlic haters will love.

ROASTED POTATO STICKS

Many healthful cookbooks have a similar recipe, but I've included one just in case you don't know the secret to healthy potatoes that taste as good as fries.

1 pound small red potatoes
Olive oil or canola oil cooking spray
Salt and freshly ground black pepper to taste

1. Preheat the oven to 450° F. Scrub the potatoes and cut them into small sticks. (The potatoes do not have to be peeled unless they are green under the skin.)

2. Spray the potatoes and a heavy baking sheet with olive oil spray; sprinkle the potatoes with salt and pepper, if desired.

3. Roast the potatoes on the lower rack of the oven for 10 minutes; remove the baking sheet from the oven, and turn the potatoes so the browned bottoms are facing up.

4. Reduce the oven temperature to 375° F; roast about 15 minutes more. Serve immediately.

MAKES 4 SERVINGS

110 calories per serving, 2 g protein, 1 g fat (0.1 sat), 24 g carbohydrate, 6 mg sodium, 443 mg potassium, 3 g dietary fiber

Exchanges: 1½ Starch

ROASTED CARROTS AND GREEN BEANS

The trick to roasting more than one vegetable at a time is to cut them into similarly sized pieces so their cooking time is the same. To cut carrots into sticks, first cut them diagonally into wedges and then into sticks.

4 large cloves garlic

2 medium carrots, cut into sticks the size of the green beans

1 pound fresh green beans, cleaned and trimmed

2 teaspoons olive oil

2 teaspoons balsamic vinegar

1. Preheat the oven to 450° F.

2. Peel the garlic cloves, and crush them by pressing down firmly with the wide part of a large kitchen knife.

3. Toss the vegetables with the olive oil and vinegar and spread evenly in a large baking sheet.

4. Roast for 10 minutes; loosen and turn vegetables; then reduce the oven temperature to 350° F, and roast until the vegetables are lightly brown and tender, about 15 minutes more.

MAKES 4 SERVINGS

85 calories per serving, 3 g protein, 3 g fat (0.3 sat), 14 g carbohydrate, 17 mg sodium, 468 mg potassium, 3 g dietary fiber

Exchanges: 2 Vegetable, 1 Fat

SPINACH SALAD

Tempering red onions in a viniagrette dressing makes them less harsh.

½ small red onion, thinly sliced

2 tablespoons Basic Dressing (page 132)

2 tablespoons chopped pecans

6 cups fresh spinach, stemmed and rinsed

1 roasted red bell pepper (from a jar), chopped

1. Place the onion in a small bowl; spoon the Basic Dressing over it.

2. Toast the pecans in a dry skillet over medium heat, stirring, until fragrant, about 5 minutes. Cool.

3. Toss the spinach, pecans, and pepper in a serving bowl with the onion and dressing. Serve immediately.

MAKES 4 SERVINGS

80 calories per serving, 3 g protein, 5 g fat (0.6 sat), 6 g carbohydrate, 78 mg sodium, 535 mg potassium, 3 g fiber

Exchanges: I Vegetable, I Fat

Variation

♥ Substitute fresh arugula for some or all of the spinach.

ZESTY THREE BEAN SALAD

Horseradish gives this three bean salad a subtle kick; use more if you like.

1 (10-ounce) package frozen green beans

1 (15½-ounce) can chickpeas, drained and rinsed

1 (15½-ounce) can red kidney beans, drained and rinsed

1 small red onion, chopped

1 medium green bell pepper, chopped

1 lime

4 tablespoons Basic Dressing (page 132)

3 tablespoons prepared horseradish sauce

1. Steam the frozen green beans in a vegetable steamer for about 5 minutes; set aside to cool.

continued

2. Combine the chickpeas, kidney beans, green beans, onion, and pepper in a large mixing bowl.

3. Cut the lime in half and squeeze the juice into a small bowl. Add the Basic Dressing and horseradish sauce.

4. Toss the dressing mixture with the beans and serve.

MAKES 8 SERVINGS

170 calories per serving, 8 g protein, 4 g fat (0.5 sat), 26 g carbohydrate, 380 mg sodium, 424 mg potassium, 3 g dietary fiber

Exchanges: I Vegetable, I ½ Starch, I Fat

BLACK BEANS AND RICE SALAD

This is a great way to have black beans and rice to go. Make it the night before for lunch the next day.

1 lime

2 tablespoons Basic Dressing (page 132)

1 (15½-ounce) can black beans, drained and rinsed

1 cup cooked brown rice

1 small red bell pepper, chopped

1 small yellow onion, chopped

2 tablespoons chopped green olives

1. Cut the lime in half and squeeze the juice into a small bowl. Add the Basic Dressing and mix with a fork.

2. In a medium bowl, toss the beans, rice, and vegetables with the dressing.

MAKES 4 SERVINGS

250 calories per serving, 12 g protein, 5 g fat (0.7 sat), 43 g carbohydrate, 33 mg sodium, 514 mg potassium, 5 g dietary fiber

Exchanges: I Vegetable, 2 Starch, ½ Very Lean Meat, I Fat

Variation

♥ Roasted garlic is a great addition if you happen to have made some for another recipe; raw garlic is a little too overpowering.

OVEN-BRAISED CARROTS AND GREEN ONIONS

Cooking carrots on top of the stove and then finishing them in the oven makes them so incredibly delicious that I often make a double batch to keep everyone happy.

2 teaspoons olive oil

4 large carrots, peeled and cut diagonally into ¼-inch slices

4 green onions, chopped

¼ cup reduced-sodium chicken broth, defatted

1. Preheat the oven to 400° F. Heat the oil over low heat in a medium skillet with an ovenproof handle. Cook the carrots and green onions for about 5 minutes, until the carrots begin to brown slightly. Add the chicken broth and bring to a boil.

2. Place the skillet in the oven until the carrots are tender, about 15 minutes.

MAKES 4 SERVINGS

55 calories per serving, 1 g protein, 2 g fat (0.3 sat), 8 g carbohydrate, 65 mg sodium, 246 mg potassium, 2 g dietary fiber

Exchanges: 1 ½ Vegetable, ½ Fat

TIP

A cast-iron skillet is perfect for going from the top of the stove into the oven. If your skillet does not have an ovenproof handle, you can protect it by wrapping the handle in heavy-duty aluminum foil.

LEMONY ROASTED ASPARAGUS

....

Roasted asparagus spears don't look as pretty as steamed, but the flavor is worth it.

> 1 lemon
> 1 pound fresh asparagus, woody stems removed
> 2 teaspoons olive oil

1. Preheat the oven to 425° F.

2. Wash and dry the outside of the lemon. Make 2 teaspoons of lemon zest by grating the yellow outside peel with the fine side of a cheese grater. Wrap the lemon in plastic wrap and refrigerate for another use.

3. Toss the asparagus spears in a shallow dish with the lemon zest and olive oil.

4. Spread the asparagus in a heavy baking sheet; roast for 15 minutes. Halfway through the cooking time, stir the asparagus to ensure even roasting. The asparagus are done when they are browned and slightly shriveled.

MAKES 4 SERVINGS

50 calories per serving, 3 g protein, 3 g fat (0.4 sat), 5 g carbohydrate, 5 mg sodium, 353 mg potassium, I g dietary fiber

Exchanges: I Vegetable, ½ Fat

Variation

♥ Omit the lemon zest for plain roasted asparagus, which is also very good.

ROASTED ACORN SQUASH

....

A couple of summers ago, the acorn squash went wild in my garden; so of course, I tried roasting it. Now it's a family favorite.

> 1 small acorn squash, seeds and pulp removed
> Olive oil cooking spray

⅛ teaspoon grated nutmeg

⅛ teaspoon salt

⅛ teaspoon freshly ground black pepper

1. Preheat the oven to 400° F. Cut the acorn squash into thin slices, about ⅛ inch thick. (Try to make the slices even or the thinner ones will cook too quickly and burn.)

2. Spray a heavy baking sheet with olive oil cooking spray; place the squash on the baking sheet. Spray each slice lightly and evenly.

3. Combine the nutmeg, salt, and pepper in a small bowl. Sprinkle each slice with a tiny pinch of the seasoning.

4. Roast for 10 minutes, loosening and turning the squash halfway through the cooking time to ensure even roasting. The squash is done when it is browned at the edges.

MAKES 4 SERVINGS

50 calories per serving, 1 g protein, 2 g fat (0.3 sat), 8 g carbohydrate, 68 mg sodium, 225 mg potassium, 1 g dietary fiber

Exchanges: ½ Starch, ½ Fat

TIP
Cooking spray is used in this recipe because the slices of squash have a large surface area and spraying allows for a thin, even coat. The nutrition analysis includes a total of 2 teaspoons olive oil.

VEGETABLE ANTIPASTO

This is a great make-ahead recipe because unlike lettuce salads, it improves with time. I like to have it for supper one night and take the leftovers to work the next day. It's also a wonderful cold dish for potluck.

4 teaspoons olive oil

2 garlic cloves

continued

2 cups cauliflower florets

¼ cup balsamic vinegar

1 (7-ounce) jar roasted red peppers, drained

½ cup pitted black olives

1 (7½-ounce) can chickpeas, drained and rinsed

1 small red onion, thinly sliced

1 teaspoon dried basil

½ teaspoon dried thyme

1. Heat 1 teaspoon of the olive oil in a large heavy skillet over medium heat; add the garlic and cauliflower and cook briefly, about 1 minute. Add the vinegar; bring to a simmer. Reduce the heat to low, cover, and cook until the cauliflower is crisp-tender, about 4 minutes.

2. Transfer the cauliflower mixture to a large bowl; add the peppers, olives, chickpeas, onion, basil, thyme, and the remaining 3 teaspoons of olive oil; toss well to combine. Refrigerate for at least 2 hours; bring to room temperature before serving.

MAKES 8 SERVINGS

80 calories per serving, 2 g protein, 4 g fat (0.7 sat), 10 g carbohydrate, 140 mg sodium, 194 mg potassium, 3 g dietary fiber

Exchanges: 2 Vegetable, 1 Fat

RUTH'S SECRET: CARAMELIZED ONIONS

About two years ago, we at *Eating Well* magazine had the good fortune of convincing cookbook author Ruth Cousineau to come work for us. We have had many incredibly talented cooks in our test kitchen before, but I have never met anyone like Ruth, who, at a moment's notice, can put together the best food I have ever tasted.

One day, Ruth and I were talking about how we ate when we were growing up, and she told me that her mother could take just about anything out of the refrigerator, cook it up, and make it taste good. (Why was I not surprised?) "Her secret," said Ruth, "was caramelized onions." Well, there it was—slow-cooked onions were also key to the great taste of Ruth's cooking, particularly her vegetarian dishes. Since then, my husband has asked me what I have been doing to make our food taste better.

Caramelized onions are used in Artichoke Hearts and Caramelized Onions (below) and in many other recipes in this book; they may also be added to bread or roll recipes or used as a topping for pizza.

1 teaspoon olive oil
1 yellow onion, thinly sliced

Heat the oil in a heavy medium skillet over medium heat. Add the onion, and cook slowly, stirring occasionally, until light golden brown, about 10 minutes.

ARTICHOKE HEARTS AND CARAMELIZED ONIONS

The name sounds fancy, but it's basically just canned artichoke hearts and slow-cooked onions. It's quite tart, so I serve it as a relish.

1 tablespoon olive oil
1 large yellow onion, thinly sliced
2 garlic cloves, minced
1 (14-ounce) can artichoke hearts, drained and quartered
¼ cup frozen lemon juice, thawed, or freshly squeezed

1. Heat the olive oil over medium-low heat in a large heavy skillet, and cook the onion, stirring occasionally, until it is light golden brown, about 10 minutes. Add the garlic and cook about 1 minute longer.

2. Add the artichoke hearts and lemon juice, cover and simmer for 5 minutes. Serve warm or refrigerate to serve as a cold marinated salad.

MAKES 4 SERVINGS

85 calories per serving, 3 g protein, 4 g fat (0.5 sat), 12 g carbohydrate, 61 mg sodium, 310 mg potassium, 1 g dietary fiber

Exchanges: 2 Vegetable, 1 Fat

Variation

♥ Balsamic vinegar may be substituted for the lemon juice, which makes the vegetables a little less tart.

ROASTED PLUM TOMATOES

Here's a good example of how roasting turns a few simple ingredients into something wonderful.

  Olive or canola oil cooking spray
  4 plum tomatoes
  1 tablespoon olive oil
  ¼ teaspoon dried basil
  ¼ teaspoon dried oregano

1. Preheat the oven to 425° F. Spray a small baking pan with cooking spray.

2. Cut the tomatoes in half and place them cut side up in the baking pan. Drizzle them with the olive oil, and roast for about 25 minutes. Sprinkle the tomatoes with the herbs, and continue to roast until their skins begin to brown, about 10 minutes longer.

MAKES 4 SERVINGS

50 calories per serving, 0 g protein, 4 g fat (0.05 sat), 4 g carbohydrate, 8 mg sodium, 204 mg potassium, 1 g dietary fiber

Exchanges: 1 Vegetable, 1 Fat

♥

CHAPTER 14

Meat-Free Entrées

These meatless main dishes are not your typical vegetarian fare. The recipes are much easier to prepare than the ones you find in most vegetarian cookbooks. And instead of relying on butter, cheese, or excessive oil for flavor, the recipes in this chapter pay strict attention to calories and saturated fat.

So where does the flavor come from? Sweet carmelized onions, garlic, bits of intensely flavored feta cheese, olives, roasted vegetables, and nuts. But to be truly good, meat-free entrées have to satisfy, so you don't fall prey to the Chinese-food trap of feeling starved an hour later. The trick to making these dishes satisfying is that each one relies on one or more "meaty" ingredients, such as mushrooms, eggplant, nuts, beans, and judicious amounts of cheese. For example, Braised Cabbage and Bulgur (page 157), an old vegetarian standby, is quite filling, yet it just doesn't feel complete without chopped peanuts to round it out. Similarly, Roasted Vegetables and Pasta (page 148) gets its staying power from chickpeas, a type of bean.

Because I'm very much aware of the general perception that vegetarian recipes take too much time to prepare, I made a special effort to make the recipes here as quick and easy as possible. Lentils and Bulgur with Walnuts (page 157), which calls for canned lentil soup and frozen greens, is ready in under thirty minutes. And my easy version of *huevos rancheros*—the tastiest egg dish ever created—takes just twenty minutes start to finish.

The most time-consuming dishes are the pizza recipes, which include directions for homemade crust. But you can also use frozen pizza crust or pizza dough, which cuts the preparation time to about thirty minutes.

ROASTED VEGETABLES AND PASTA

The beauty of this dish is its simplicity. All of the vegetables are roasted together and tossed with the pasta in the roasting pan.

10 garlic cloves, peeled
4 ripe plum tomatoes, halved and quartered
1 small eggplant, peeled and cut into cubes
1 large red bell pepper, seeded and cut into strips
1 medium yellow onion, sliced
1 (7½-ounce) can chickpeas, drained and rinsed
1 tablespoon olive oil
1 teaspoon dried basil
½ pound ziti
1 tablespoon balsamic vinegar

1. Preheat the oven to 450° F; set the pasta water to boil.

2. Toss the garlic and vegetables with the olive oil and basil in a large shallow roasting pan.

3. Set the roasting pan on the lower rack of the oven and roast for 20 minutes, stirring every 5 minutes to ensure even roasting.

4. Meanwhile, cook the ziti according to the package directions. Add the cooked, drained ziti to the roasting pan, with the balsamic vinegar, and toss with the roasted vegetables to mix. Transfer to a platter and serve.

MAKES 4 SERVINGS

335 calories per serving, 11 g protein, 6 g fat (0.8 sat), 61 g carbohydrate, 210 mg sodium, 500 mg potassium, 5 g dietary fiber

Exchanges: 3 Vegetable, 2½ Starch, ½ Very Lean Meat, 1 Fat

MED-MEX CASSEROLE

This one-dish entrée seems too easy to be so good. The key to its great flavor is sautéing the vegetables before baking.

2 teaspoons olive oil

1 medium onion

1 medium zucchini, cut into matchsticks

1 medium bell pepper, seeded and chopped

2 garlic cloves, minced

1 (15-ounce) can black beans, drained and rinsed

1 cup frozen corn kernels

4 (6-inch) frozen corn tortillas, thawed

1 (10-ounce) jar prepared salsa

4 ounces shredded reduced-fat Cheddar cheese

1. Preheat the oven to 350° F. Heat the oil in a large nonstick skillet and cook the onion, zucchini, and pepper over medium heat, stirring, until soft, about 5 minutes. Add the garlic, beans, and corn; cook, stirring, about 3 minutes.

2. Arrange the tortillas in a small lasagna pan. Spread the cooked vegetables over the tortillas, top with the salsa and then with the cheese. Bake for 25 minutes, until the cheese is melted.

MAKES 4 SERVINGS

380 calories per serving, 23 g protein, 11 g fat (0.4 sat), 56 g carbohydrate, 393 mg sodium, 875 mg potassium, 8 g dietary fiber

Exchanges: 1 Vegetable, 3 Starch, 1½ Lean Meat, 1 Fat

CANNED CANCER PROTECTION

If you've ever grown and canned your own tomatoes, you know how many tomatoes it takes. Canned tomato products are a great bargain! But you may not know that tomatoes also protect against cancer. They contain lycopene, the plant pigment that gives them their red color, which is an antioxidant cousin of beta-carotene that has been associated with powerful cancer protection, particularly against prostate cancer. Interestingly, lycopene is not destroyed by canning; in fact, the heat of processing releases lycopene from the plant cells and makes it more available to the body. And tomato products, like sauce and tomato paste, are very high in lycopene because they are concentrated sources of tomatoes. This means that you get more lycopene from tomato sauce than you do from a fresh tomato.

EGGPLANT PARMESAN

In most recipes for eggplant Parmesan, the eggplant is fried in oil; and if you've ever done this, you know that eggplant soaks up oil like a sponge. In this version, slices of eggplant are prebaked with a light coating of oil, which makes them melt-in-your-mouth good and reduces the calories to about a third of the original.

    1 large or 2 small eggplants (1 pound)
    Salt
    1 recipe Easy Tomato Sauce (page 164)
    Olive oil cooking spray
    ½ cup freshly grated Parmesan cheese
    2 teaspoons dried oregano

1. Peel and thinly slice the eggplant. Salt the slices and put them in a large colander placed over a plate to drain off their bitter juices. The eggplant should drain for at least 30 minutes.

2. Preheat the oven to 400° F. Prepare the Easy Tomato Sauce. Spray a heavy baking sheet with olive oil.

3. Wipe the eggplant slices with a paper towel to remove the salt and excess liquid. Place the slices on the baking sheet and spray the tops with olive oil. Sprinkle each slice with a small amount of Parmesan cheese, saving more than half of the cheese for the topping.

4. Reduce the oven temperature to 350° F. Bake until the tops just begin to turn golden, 12 to 15 minutes. Spread half the tomato sauce on the bottom of a casserole dish, and layer the eggplant slices. Top with the remaining tomato sauce, the oregano, and the remaining cheese. Bake for 20 minutes or until the casserole is bubbly and cheese is lightly browned.

MAKES 4 SERVINGS

175 calories per serving, 10 g protein, 6 g fat (3 sat), 24 g carbohydrate, 704 mg sodium, 977 mg potassium, 6 g dietary fiber

Exchanges: 3 Vegetable, 1 Lean Meat, 1 Fat

TIP

Leftover Eggplant Parmesan makes a great sandwich filling.

VEGETABLE PIE

I keep a bag of frozen broccoli on hand to use in this recipe and in omelets because it is quick, easy, and just as nutritious as fresh.

Olive oil cooking spray

1 tablespoon olive oil

1 large onion, chopped

10 ounces fresh mushrooms, sliced

1 garlic clove, chopped

2 large eggs

½ cup part-skim ricotta cheese

½ cup skim milk

5 sun-dried tomatoes, cut into thin strips (page 105)

1 (10-ounce) package chopped frozen broccoli, thawed

1 teaspoon dried basil

continued

1. Preheat the oven to 350° F. Lightly spray a 10-inch quiche or pie pan with cooking spray.

2. Heat the olive oil in a large nonstick skillet and cook the onion and mushrooms over medium heat, stirring, until their liquid has evaporated, about 5 minutes. Add the garlic, and cook briefly; remove the vegetables to the prepared pan.

3. Beat the eggs in a medium bowl and add the ricotta and milk. Pour the mixture over the onion and mushrooms. Stir in the tomatoes, broccoli, and basil. Bake for 30 minutes, until set. Cool slightly, cut into wedges, and serve.

MAKES 4 SERVINGS

180 calories per serving, 12 g protein, 9 g fat (2.8 sat), 15 g carbohydrate, 110 mg sodium, 610 mg potassium, 4 g dietary fiber

Exchanges: 3 Vegetables, 1 Lean Meat, 1 Fat

SPINACH PIE

....

This is my version of Greek spanakopita, which can be served hot or cold. Lightly spraying the phyllo sheets with olive oil allows you to keep the fat and calories lower than traditional spanakopita, which calls for brushing each layer with oil or melted butter.

Olive oil cooking spray
1 teaspoon olive oil
1 large onion, chopped
2 cloves garlic, minced
1 (10-ounce) package chopped spinach, thawed
4 ounces feta cheese, crumbled
1 (16-ounce) container low-fat cottage cheese
2 teaspoons dried oregano
4 ounces refrigerated phyllo dough (⅓ package)

1. Preheat the oven to 350° F. Spray a 9-inch square baking dish with olive oil.

2. Heat the 1 teaspoon oil in a large nonstick skillet and cook the onion over medium heat, stirring, for about 5 minutes. Add the garlic, and cook for about 1 minute. Add the spinach, and cook briefly, until the spinach is fairly dry. Turn off the heat; mix in the feta, cottage cheese, and oregano.

3. To prepare the phyllo, moisten a clean kitchen towel with water, unfold the dough and cover it with the towel to keep it from drying out.

4. Place one sheet of phyllo, folded in half, on the bottom of the pan; spray lightly with oil. Keeping the unused phyllo covered, place another folded sheet in the pan and spray; repeat until you have used 5 sheets of phyllo.

5. Spoon the cheese-spinach mixture over the phyllo layers and spread evenly. Repeat Step 4, adding 5 more folded phyllo sheets for the top crust. Lightly spray the top of the pie; bake for 30 minutes, until the edges begin to brown. Cool slightly and cut into 9 squares.

MAKES 9 SERVINGS

205 calories per serving, 16 g protein, 6 g fat (3.4 sat), 20 g carbohydrate, 662 mg sodium, 272 mg potassium, 1 g dietary fiber

Exchanges: 1 Vegetable, 1 Starch, 1½ Lean Meat

TIPS

♥ *Look for fresh refrigerated phyllo dough so you can use what you need and freeze the leftovers. If you can find only frozen, you will have to defrost the entire package and refreeze the leftovers.*

♥ *If the spinach is not completely thawed, run under cold water and then press out the excess water.*

GREEK PIZZA

I usually make my pizza dough in the morning and let it rise in a cool place until I come home from work. A large Greek pizza with salad and wine is great when friends come over for a casual dinner. If you want to make only one pizza, freeze half the dough for another time.

FOR THE CRUST

2 teaspoons active dry yeast

½ teaspoon sugar

1 cup warm water

1 teaspoon olive oil

2 cups unbleached bread flour

½ cup whole wheat flour

½ teaspoon salt

FOR THE TOPPING

1 teaspoon olive oil

1 small yellow onion, thinly sliced

1 recipe Easy Tomato Sauce (page 164)

1 cup frozen spinach, thawed

10 good-quality black olives, pitted and chopped

1 roasted red pepper (from a jar), chopped

½ cup crumbled feta cheese

½ cup shredded part-skim mozzarella cheese

1 tablespoon dried oregano

1. Make the crust. In a medium bowl, stir the yeast, sugar, and water together; let sit until foamy, about 5 minutes.

2. Stir in the olive oil; add the flours, ½ cup at a time, and then add the salt. Mix by hand until all the lumps are gone.

3. Turn the dough out onto a floured surface and knead until it is satiny and stretchy, 8 to 10 minutes. Place the dough in an oiled bowl, cover with plastic wrap, and let it rise in a cool but draft-free spot for at least 2 hours.

4. Preheat the oven to 500° F. (If you have a pizza stone, place it in the oven before preheating.)

5. Roll or press the dough into a large heavy baking pan, such as a jelly roll pan, or into two 10- to 12-inch pizza pans.

6. Make the topping. Heat the olive oil in a large heavy skillet over medium-low heat, and cook the onion, stirring, until it is golden, about 10 minutes. Cover the top of the dough evenly with the Easy Tomato Sauce, vegetables, cheeses, and oregano.

7. Bake until the cheeses are fully melted and the crust just starts to brown, 12 to 15 minutes. (One large pizza takes longer to bake than two small pizzas, which take 10 to 11 minutes each.)

MAKES 8 SERVINGS

255 calories per serving, 10 g protein, 5 g fat (2 sat), 44 g carbohydrate, 396 mg sodium, 590 mg potassium, 5 g dietary fiber

Exchanges: 2 Vegetable, 2 Starch, 1/2 Lean Meat, 1/2 Fat

Variation

♥ Other great pizza toppings include sliced mushrooms, sliced artichoke hearts, and thin slices of roasted eggplant.

`TIP`

If you are serving people with different preferences, make two pizzas so you can add and subtract toppings as desired.

PIZZA WITH CARAMELIZED ONIONS AND BLACK OLIVES

My family loves this pizza as much as the ones with lots of tomato sauce, so I often make one of each.

FOR THE CRUST

2 teaspoons active dry yeast

1/2 teaspoon sugar

1 cup warm water

continued

1 teaspoon olive oil

2 cups unbleached bread flour

½ cup whole wheat flour

½ teaspoon salt

FOR THE TOPPING

1 tablespoon olive oil

1 large yellow onion

¼ cup chopped black olives

¼ cup freshly grated Parmesan cheese

Freshly ground black pepper to taste

1. Make the crust. In a medium bowl, stir the yeast, sugar, and water together; let sit until foamy, about 5 minutes.

2. Stir in the olive oil; add the flours, ½ cup at a time; then add the salt and mix by hand until all the lumps are gone.

3. Turn the dough onto a floured surface and knead until it is satiny and stretchy, 8 to 10 minutes. Place the dough in an oiled bowl, cover with plastic wrap, and let it rise in a cool but draft-free spot for at least 2 hours.

4. Preheat the oven to 500° F. (If you have a pizza stone, place it in the oven before preheating.)

5. Roll or press the dough into a large heavy baking pan, such as a jelly roll pan, or into two 10- to12-inch pizza pans.

6. Make the topping. Heat the olive oil in a large heavy skillet over medium-low heat, and cook the onion, stirring, until it is golden, about 10 minutes. Spread the dough evenly with the caramelized onion, olives, and Parmesan. Season with pepper.

7. Bake until the edges are lightly browned and the cheese is melted, about 12 minutes for two small pizzas, 15 to 18 minutes for one large pizza.

MAKES 8 SERVINGS

200 calories per serving, 1 g protein, 4 g fat (2 sat), 34 g carbohydrate, 241 mg sodium, 119 mg potassium, 3 g dietary fiber

Exchanges: 1 Vegetable, 2 Starch, 1 Fat

BRAISED CABBAGE AND BULGUR

This dish is one of my old standbys because I usually have all the ingredients on hand, and it's so easy to fix. With some crusty whole wheat bread, supper is ready in no time.

2 teaspoons olive oil

1 large onion, chopped

¾ cup bulgur

2 cups chopped cabbage

2 medium carrots, sliced

1½ cups reduced-sodium chicken broth, defatted

½ cup chopped peanuts

1. Heat the oil in a large heavy skillet with a lid or in a Dutch oven over medium heat. Add the onion, bulgur, cabbage, and carrots, and cook until lightly browned, about 2 minutes.

2. Add the broth and bring to a boil. Reduce the heat; cover and simmer until the bulgur is tender, about 12 minutes. Top with the chopped peanuts and serve.

MAKES 4 SERVINGS

260 calories per serving, 10 g protein, 12 g fat (1.6 g sat), 33 g carbohydrate, 270 mg sodium, 524 mg potassium, 10 g dietary fiber

Exchanges: 1 Vegetable, 2 Starch, 1 Medium-Fat Meat, ½ Fat

LENTILS AND BULGUR WITH WALNUTS

This is the vegetarian version of Lentils and Bulgur with Sausage (page 170). Toasted walnuts and red pepper flakes stand in for the spicy sausage.

1 (19-ounce) can lentil soup

⅓ cup bulgur

1 cup frozen greens, such as collard, mustard, or spinach

continued

5 sun-dried tomatoes, snipped into strips

⅛ teaspoon red pepper flakes (or more to taste)

¼ cup chopped walnuts

1. Mix the lentil soup, bulgur, greens, tomatoes, and red pepper flakes in a large skillet with a cover or in a Dutch oven. Bring to a boil, reduce the heat to low, cover, and simmer for 20 minutes.

2. Meanwhile, toast the walnuts in a dry skillet over medium heat, stirring occasionally, until fragrant, about 5 minutes.

3. Top the lentil mixture with the toasted walnuts and serve.

MAKES 4 SERVINGS

180 calories per serving, 9 g protein, 6 g fat (0.3 sat), 25 g carbohydrate, 404 mg sodium, 701 mg potassium, 5 g dietary fiber

Exchanges: 1½ Starch, 1 Medium-Fat Meat

ABOUT RISOTTO

Elegant enough for entertaining, yet simple enough for a midweek supper, risotto is a creamy rice dish that relies on starch, rather than fat, for its creaminess. Risotto dishes evolved in the Mediterranean to take advantage of plump Italian rice, which develops a creamy consistency as the grain swells and absorbs liquid. With its smooth texture and mild flavor, risotto needs only a little garlic and chopped onion to make a delicious side dish. Add vegetables or seafood, and risotto becomes a satisfying meal in itself.

Risotto is easy to make, but the technique works only with plump short-grain rices such as Arborio, and it requires almost constant stirring to develop its creamy texture. Many recipes call for up to ¼ cup fat for 1 cup of uncooked rice, but 1 tablespoon olive oil is more than enough for sautéing the onion and garlic. With less added oil, there's room to stir in some flavorful Parmesan cheese before serving.

In the Mediterranean, risotto is often combined with seafood, greens, fresh herbs, and vegetables in season. If you like the risotto recipes in this chapter, you might also like to try Shrimp and Pepper Risotto (page 180).

BASIC RISOTTO

....

    2 teaspoons olive oil

    1 small yellow onion, chopped

    1 clove garlic, minced

    1 cup Arborio rice

    3 cups chicken broth or 1 (14½-ounce) can low-sodium broth,
        defatted, and diluted with water to make 3 cups liquid

1. Heat the olive oil in a large saucepan over medium heat. Add the onion and cook until soft, stirring, about 3 minutes; add the garlic, and cook briefly.

2. Add the rice, and cook for 2 minutes. Add 1 cup of the broth, stir well, and bring to a boil. Reduce the heat, and gradually stir in the rest of the broth, ½ cup at a time, cooking and stirring and adding more broth as the liquid is absorbed. The risotto is done when thick and creamy. Serve immediately.

MAKES 4 SERVINGS

210 calories per serving, 5 g protein, 3g fat (0.5 sat), 41 g carbohydrate, 275 mg sodium, 76 mg potassium, trace dietary fiber

Exchanges: 2½ Starch, ½ Fat

ZUCCHINI RISOTTO

....

    2 teaspoons olive oil

    1 small yellow onion, chopped

    1 medium zucchini, sliced across the diagonal and cut into match
        sticks

    1 clove garlic, minced

    1 cup Arborio rice

    3 cups chicken broth or 1 (14½-ounce) can low-sodium broth,
        defatted, and diluted to make 3 cups liquid

    ¼ cup freshly grated Parmesan cheese

continued

1. Heat the olive oil in a Dutch oven over medium heat. Add the onion and zucchini and cook, stirring, about 5 minutes until soft. Add the garlic and cook until fragrant, about 1 minute.

2. Add the rice, and cook for 2 minutes. Add 1 cup of the broth, stir well, and bring to a boil. Reduce the heat, and gradually stir in the rest of the broth ½ cup at a time, cooking, stirring, and adding more broth as the liquid is absorbed, until the risotto is thick and creamy. Stir in the Parmesan just before serving.

MAKES 4 SERVINGS

285 calories per serving, 9 g protein, 6 g fat (2.8 sat), 41 g carbohydrate, 648 mg sodium, 433 mg potassium, 1 g dietary fiber

Exchanges: 1 Vegetable, 2½ Starch, ½ Lean Meat

EASY HUEVOS RANCHEROS

Who says eggs aren't good for you? This easy version of Mexican-style eggs has everything a healthy meal should have, including a good boost of cancer-fighting lycopene from the salsa. This is my favorite weekend breakfast, but it is also good as a quick-and-easy supper.

Olive or canola oil cooking spray
2 (6-inch) corn tortillas
1 large egg
2 large egg whites
1 teaspoon olive oil
1 clove garlic, finely minced
½ cup canned black beans, drained and rinsed
1 cup thick salsa
¼ cup shredded low-fat Cheddar cheese

1. Preheat the oven to 350° F. Spray a small baking dish with cooking spray. Place the tortillas in the dish.

2. In a small bowl, beat the egg and egg whites together with a fork. Heat the 1 teaspoon olive oil in a large heavy skillet over medium heat. Cook the

garlic and beans for about 1 minute; add the eggs and heat, stirring, just until they begin to cook. Pour the egg mixture over the tortillas.

3. Spoon the salsa over the eggs, top with the cheese, and bake until the cheese is melted, about 12 minutes.

MAKES 2 SERVINGS

280 calories per serving, 18 g protein, 11 g fat (0.9 sat), 33 g carbohydrate, 654 mg sodium, 651 mg potassium, 3 g dietary fiber

Exchanges: 2 Starch, 2 Medium-Fat Meat

TIP

You can adjust the heat of your huevos *by using mild, medium, or hot salsa.*

♥

CHAPTER 15

Almost Vegetarian Entrées

Most of us grew up with positive feelings about red meat—it builds strong bodies, it's all-American, steak is diet food. Remember when serving prime ribs was a sure sign of success? This is why the thought of giving beef up is difficult for many people, even though we now know that consuming large amounts of meat on a regular basis raises the risk of many diet-related diseases.

But you can still enjoy a little meat without compromising your health by using it as a flavoring, rather than the center of the meal. This is a lesson we've learned from studying healthy patterns of traditional eating. In Asia, where pork, rather than beef, is usually available, small amounts are used in dishes that contain generous amounts of rice, noodles, and vegetables. In the Mediterranean, small amounts of pork preserved as prosciutto or pancetta (leaner equivalents of our ham and bacon) are used to flavor bean and pasta dishes.

Most of the recipes in this chapter evolved over the years in my own kitchen as my family gradually cut down on the meat in our diet. Little Meat Chili (page 169), for example, started out as the standard hamburger-laden version that contained more calories and fat in one serving than anyone other than a professional football player needs in an entire day. I found that braising lean round steak in broth makes the chili so good that the small bit of meat—about an ounce per person—satisfies even the heartiest appetites. In fact, I first wrote the recipe down when a friend who bears a very strong resemblance to Grizzly Adams and who loves to hunt, fish, and eat kept asking me for it so he could make it at home.

BEANS AND GREENS CASSEROLE

Beans and greens are the mainstays of the Mediterranean diet; with a bit of good Parmesan cheese and Italian turkey sausage, you have a healthy dish that's full of flavor.

1 large bunch beet greens, well washed, tough stems removed

4 teaspoons olive oil

1 clove garlic, minced

1 (14-ounce) can diced tomatoes, drained

1 (15½-ounce) can red kidney beans, drained and rinsed

½ teaspoon dried thyme

Pinch red pepper flakes

4 ounces sweet Italian turkey sausage

1 small onion, chopped

2 tablespoons plain dry bread crumbs

2 tablespoons freshly grated Parmesan cheese

1. Preheat the oven to 350° F. Stack the greens lengthwise and cut them across the grain into ribbons.

2. Heat 2 teaspoons of the olive oil in a large heavy skillet over medium heat; add the greens and garlic, and cook, stirring, about 3 to 5 minutes, until the greens are wilted. Remove to a 10-inch casserole, and add the tomatoes, beans, thyme, and red pepper flakes.

3. Add the sausage to the same skillet, and cook over medium heat, about 5 minutes, until lightly browned. Break the sausage into bite-sized pieces with a fork, and add to the casserole.

4. To make the topping, heat the remaining 2 teaspoons of olive oil over medium heat; cook the onions briefly and toss bread crumbs and cheese with

onions in the skillet. Sprinkle evenly over the bean mixture in the casserole. Bake for 30 minutes, until bread crumb topping is lightly browned.

MAKES 4 SERVINGS

240 calories per serving, 15 g protein, 8 g fat (2 sat), 28 g carbohydrate, 760 mg sodium, 917 mg potassium, 8 g dietary fiber

Exchanges: 2 Vegetable, 1 Starch, 1 Lean Meat, 1 Fat

EASY TOMATO SAUCE

There are so many jarred sauces available today that it almost doesn't seem worth it to make your own. But here's a recipe that is almost as easy as opening a jar and is far less expensive. (I always stock up on canned tomatoes in September when the price is at its lowest.) And because herbs tend to get bitter when canned, this sauce is much fresher tasting.

1 (28-ounce) can crushed tomatoes
1 bay leaf
Dried oregano or basil to taste
1 clove garlic, peeled

In a medium saucepan over medium-low heat, simmer the tomatoes with the herbs and garlic. For pizza sauce, simmer until it gets nice and thick, about 30 minutes, because a thin sauce makes the crust soggy. For other recipes simmer about 15 minutes. Remove the garlic and bay leaf before using the sauce.

MAKES 3 CUPS

55 calories per ½-cup serving, 2 g protein, 0 g fat, 13 g carbohydrate, 27 mg sodium, 558 mg potassium, 3 g dietary fiber

Exchanges: 2 Vegetable

TIP
Use fresh herbs when they're available.

BAKED STUFFED PEPPERS

Thin-skinned peppers work best because they leave more room for the filling. Green peppers are fine; but if you can get red peppers at a reasonable price, they are even better.

1 medium eggplant

Salt

4 medium bell peppers, seeded and halved

1 recipe Easy Tomato Sauce (page 164)

1 teaspoon olive oil

10 ounces mushrooms, sliced

1 large onion, chopped

½ pound lean ground beef

¼ cup green olives, pitted and chopped

¾ cup cooked brown rice

½ cup shredded reduced-fat Cheddar cheese

1. Preheat the oven to 350° F. Peel and cube the eggplant. Place it in a colander, place colander over a plate, salt lightly, and let the juices drain while preparing the other ingredients.

2. Blanch the peppers in boiling water for 3 minutes; drain and dry them. Spread the Easy Tomato Sauce in a lasagna pan and arrange the drained peppers open side up in the sauce. Wipe the eggplant with a paper towel to remove the salt and juices.

3. Heat the oil in a large heavy skillet over medium heat, and cook the mushrooms, eggplant, and onion, stirring, until the mushrooms begin to release their juices, about 5 minutes; remove the vegetables from the skillet and set aside.

4. Add the beef to the skillet, and cook over medium heat until browned. Place the meat in a colander and rinse with hot water to drain off the fat. Put the mushrooms, onion, and eggplant back into the skillet; add the meat, olives, and rice, and toss to mix.

5. Spoon the filling into the pepper halves; top each with cheese. Bake until the cheese is completely melted and begins to brown, about 30 minutes.

MAKES 8 SERVINGS

172 calories per serving, 13 g protein, 5 g fat (1.5 sat), 22g carbohydrate, 230 mg sodium, 792 mg potassium, 5 g dietary fiber

Exchanges: 3 Vegetable, ½ Starch, 1 Medium-Fat Meat

SEEING RED

Mediterranean cooks use red bell peppers exclusively, because to them a green pepper is unripe. Well, they do have a point. If left on the vine, bell peppers mature to the bright red stage, which makes them not only sweeter but more nutritious. As you might guess from its color, a red pepper has ten times the amount of carotenoids as does a green pepper, including not only beta-carotene but also lutein and zeaxanthin, the two carotenoids that protect the eyes against macular degeneration, the leading cause of blindness in people over 65. (Greens are another excellent source of these two carotenoids.) Granted, fresh red peppers are almost always more expensive than green, but they're worth it. Here's a tip: When you're shopping, check out the roasted red peppers in a jar (page 105), and stock up when you see them at a good price. The canning process does not destroy carotenoids, and you can use them in place of fresh peppers in salads and many recipes.

RED BEANS AND RICE

The secret to this flavorful dish is cooking the onions over low heat until they turn golden and very sweet, which is a nice foil to the hot, smoky chipotle peppers. If you like it hot, use two or more peppers.

¾ cup long-grain brown rice
1 tablespoon olive oil
2 large onions, sliced
3 ounces Canadian bacon, chopped
2 cloves garlic, minced
1 canned chipotle pepper
1 (15½-can) dark red kidney beans, drained and rinsed

½ cup canned crushed tomatoes

1 bay leaf

1. Prepare the rice according to the package directions.

2. Meanwhile, heat the oil in a large heavy skillet over low heat. Add the onions, and cook, stirring occasionally, until golden, about 15 minutes. Add the Canadian bacon and garlic, and cook, stirring, for about 2 minutes.

3. Add the pepper, beans, tomatoes, and bay leaf. Simmer over low heat for about 10 minutes. Remove the bay leaf and serve the beans over the rice.

MAKES 4 SERVINGS

275 calories per serving, 15 g protein, 6 g fat (1 sat), 42 g carbohydrate, 256 mg sodium, 692 mg potassium, 5 g dietary fiber

Exchanges: 1½ Vegetable, 2 Starch, 1 Lean Meat, ½ Fat

VEGETABLE LASAGNA WITH A BIT OF SAUSAGE

With its tightly packed layers of full-fat cheese, ground beef, and noodles, the lasagna we once all knew and loved is about as dense in calories and saturated fat as you can get. But you don't have to give up this wonderful dish forever. Here's an updated version with all the taste and a fraction of the fat and calories.

32 ounces low-fat cottage cheese

2 teaspoons olive oil

10 ounces mushrooms, chopped

4 ounces low-fat Italian turkey sausage, sliced

6 cups (2 recipes) Easy Tomato Sauce (page 164)

12 lasagna noodles

12 ounces skim milk ricotta cheese

1 (10-ounce) package chopped frozen spinach, thawed and drained

1 cup shredded part-skim mozzarella cheese

continued

1. Place the cottage cheese in a colander over a bowl; set aside, and let the liquid drain. Begin heating the water for the lasagna noodles. Preheat the oven to 350° F.

2. Heat the oil in a large nonstick skillet over medium heat, and cook the mushrooms and sausage, stirring, until the mushrooms begin to turn golden, about 5 minutes. In a large bowl, combine the mushroom mixture with the Easy Tomato Sauce.

3. Cook the lasagna noodles for only about 5 minutes. (They will be floppy, but they shouldn't fall apart.)

4. Mix the cottage cheese, ricotta, and spinach together in a large bowl.

5. Just cover the bottom of a lasagna pan with the sauce mixture; then layer the other ingredients as follows: 4 lasagna noodles, half the cheese mixture, one-third of the remaining sauce, 4 lasagna noodles, the rest of the cheese mixture, one-half of the remaining sauce, 4 lasagna noodles, and the remaining sauce.

6. Bake for 25 minutes; sprinkle the top with the mozzarella, and bake until the cheese melts, about 10 minutes more. Let cool slightly, slice, and serve.

MAKES 12 SERVINGS

290 calories per serving, 22 g protein, 7 g fat (2 sat), 38 g carbohydrate, 400 mg sodium, 920 mg potassium, 4 g dietary fiber

Exchanges: 2 Vegetable, 2 Starch, 2 Medium-Fat Meat

Variations

◊ Two (28-ounce) jars of tomato sauce may be substituted for the home-made; but if the sauce is thin, you may have to simmer it for 15 or 20 minutes to thicken it.

◊ Chopped frozen broccoli may be substituted for the spinach.

LITTLE MEAT CHILI

A small amount of lean round steak goes a long way to give this chili the flavor of the fatty meaty chilis we have all known and loved. The recipe is generous because chili is a great party food and it tastes even better the next day.

1 pound round steak, partially frozen

1 tablespoon olive oil

2 large onions, chopped

2 cloves garlic, minced

1 (14½-ounce) can reduced-sodium beef broth, defatted

1 cup dry red table wine

1 (14-ounce) can of diced tomatoes

12 sun-dried tomatoes, snipped into strips

1 (15½-ounce) can black beans, drained and rinsed

1 (15½-ounce) can pinto beans, drained and rinsed

2 (15½-ounce) cans dark red kidney beans, drained and rinsed

1 chopped chipotle pepper (page 99)

2 teaspoons dried oregano

20 stuffed green olives, sliced into circles

1. Slice the steak across the grain into thin slices.

2. Heat the oil in a large Dutch oven over medium heat, and cook the meat with the onions until both are nicely browned. Add the garlic and cook briefly; add the broth, and bring to a boil; reduce the heat to medium-low, cover, and simmer for 15 minutes. Add the wine, both kinds of tomatoes, beans, pepper, and oregano; cover and simmer for 60 minutes. Uncover the pot after 45 minutes to check the liquid level; if the chili looks too watery, cook uncovered for the last 15 minutes.

3. Stir in the chopped olives just before serving.

MAKES 12 SERVINGS

295 calories per serving, 23 g protein, 5 g fat (1 sat), 39 g carbohydrate, 255 mg sodium, 896 mg potassium, 5 g dietary fiber

Exchanges: 2 Vegetable, 2 Starch, 1½ Lean Meat

LENTILS AND BULGUR WITH SAUSAGE

This one-skillet dish was inspired by a similar recipe developed by Ruth Cousineau for *Eating Well* magazine using pantry items, like lentil soup and bulgur, to make a quick-and-easy meal.

1 (19-ounce) can lentil soup

⅓ cup bulgur

1 cup frozen greens, such as collard or spinach, unthawed

5 sun-dried tomatoes, cut into strips

4 ounces hot Italian turkey sausage

1. Mix the lentil soup, bulgur, frozen spinach, and tomatoes in a large skillet with a cover or in a Dutch oven. Cook over medium heat for 20 minutes.

2. Meanwhile, brown the sausage in a small skillet over medium heat. Break the sausage into bite-sized pieces with a fork. Add to the other ingredients, stir, cover, and continue cooking for the remaining time.

MAKES 4 SERVINGS

195 calories per serving, 15 g protein, 4 g fat (1 sat), 25 g carbohydrate, 763 mg sodium, 740 mg potassium, 4 g dietary fiber

Exchanges: 1½ Starch, 2 Very Lean Meat

FRITTATA

Frittatas are considered supper food around our house, particularly in the summer when we are always looking for ways to make a meal of garden vegetables.

1 tablespoon olive oil

1 small potato, very thinly sliced

1 medium onion, chopped

2 ounces proscuitto or thinly sliced lean ham, chopped

1 small zucchini, thinly sliced

4 large eggs

2 large egg whites

¼ cup freshly grated Parmesan cheese

1. Heat the oil in a medium skillet with a broiler-proof handle over medium heat. Add the potato and onion, and cook, stirring, about 5 minutes. (Add a little water to the skillet if the potato begins to stick.) Add the prosciutto and zucchini; and cook 5 minutes.

2. Preheat the broiler. Beat the eggs and egg whites together in a large bowl with a fork. Pour the egg mixture over the vegetables and cook the egg mixture, gently lifting it around the edges with a spatula to let the uncooked egg run to the bottom of the skillet. When the bottom is set, sprinkle the cheese on top. Place the skillet under the broiler until the cheese is melted, about 4 minutes.

MAKES 4 SERVINGS

215 calories per serving, 15 g protein, 11 g fat (3.6 sat), 12 g carbohydrate, 387 mg sodium, 395 mg potassium, 2 g dietary fiber

Exchanges: 1 Vegetable, ½ Starch, 2 Lean Meat, 1 Fat

Variations

ᴠ Other frittata fixings include sliced mushrooms, chopped peppers, fresh spinach or other greens, chopped plum tomatoes, and artichoke hearts.

RED LENTIL AND RICE SOUP

Red lentils are lighter and less meaty tasting than brown lentils, and they're just as nutritious.

1 tablespoon olive oil

¼ teaspoon ground cumin

1 medium onion, chopped

1 celery rib, chopped

continued

1 medium carrot

4 ounces Canadian bacon, chopped

2 cloves garlic, minced

¾ cup dried red lentils, picked over and rinsed

¼ cup long-grain brown rice

1 (14-ounce) can diced tomatoes

1 (14½-ounce) can low-sodium chicken broth, defatted

4 cups water

1 bay leaf

Chopped fresh parsley leaves for garnish

Heat the olive oil in a 5-quart saucepan over medium heat. Add the cumin and cook briefly, stirring; add the celery and carrot, and cook, stirring, for about 4 minutes. Add the bacon and garlic, and cook, stirring, another 2 minutes. Add the remaining ingredients, except the parsley, and bring to a boil; reduce the heat to low, cover, and simmer for 45 minutes. Remove the bay leaf, garnish with the parsley, and serve.

MAKES 4 SERVINGS

210 calories per serving, 14 g protein, 6 g fat (1.1 sat), 27 g carbohydrate, 664 mg sodium, 602 mg potassium, 5 g dietary fiber

Exchanges: 2 Vegetable, 1 Starch, 1½ Lean Meat

YELLOW SPLIT PEA SOUP

Yes, this is so easy that once you've made it, you won't need a recipe. Don't forget how good this soup is for you!

½ pound dried split yellow peas, picked over and rinsed

5 cups water

3 medium carrots, chopped

1 small potato, cut into small chunks

1 medium onion, thinly sliced

2 large cloves garlic, peeled and crushed

2 teaspoons dried rosemary

3 ounces prosciutto or lean ham, finely diced

2 cups reduced-sodium chicken broth, defatted

1. Place the peas and water in a large saucepan and bring to a boil.

2. Reduce the heat to medium-low; add the remaining ingredients. Cover and simmer for 2 hours. Add more water if the soup gets too thick.

3. Remove the garlic cloves before serving.

MAKES 6 SERVINGS

190 calories per serving, 15 g protein, 2 g fat (0.5 sat), 30 g carbohydrate, 449 mg sodium, 644 mg potassium, 2 g dietary fiber

Exchanges: I Vegetable, I ½ Starch, I Very Lean Meat

CHAPTER 16

♥

Poultry and Seafood Entrées

Everyone knows that chicken and fish are good for you; and this is one nutritional belief that couldn't be more true, particularly for people with type 2 diabetes. There's nothing like perfectly cooked chicken or turkey breast or a nice piece of fish when you really need a good meal. As long as you choose a healthy recipe, there's no worry about your blood sugar or blood fats.

To me—the short-cut queen of cooking from scratch—skinless, boneless chicken and turkey breasts are modern-day wonders. When I think about what it takes to remove the skin and bones from those birds so that we can have pure lean protein to cook with, I am certainly thankful that I don't live back in the good old days.

Even though I don't cook fish as much as I should, I do appreciate the fact that I can live in Vermont and still have salmon, shrimp, or haddock almost any time. I prefer preparing frozen fish, which is just as nutritious as fresh, to avoid the unpleasant experience of having the smell of fish permeate the house for days. Fresh salmon, however, isn't usually a problem, which is a good thing, because it is the ultimate source of omega-3s and is a fish everyone loves. And don't forget canned albacore tuna—it's also a good source of omega-3s, it's convenient, and you can pack it to go.

CHICKEN CACCIATORE

....

Cacciatore, or hunters' stew, was traditionally made with wild game, such as rabbit. In this version, the chicken thighs become meltingly tender in the flavorful vegetable stew.

1 tablespoon olive oil

1 pound skinless, boneless chicken thighs

2 medium yellow onions

1 pound mushrooms, sliced

1 small zucchini, sliced

1 celery rib, sliced

2 carrots, finely chopped

1 (28-ounce) can tomatoes

2 tablespoons tomato paste

1 clove garlic, minced

¾ cup dry red wine

1 teaspoon dried rosemary

1. Heat the oil in a Dutch oven over medium-high heat; add the chicken and brown well on both sides.

2. Remove the chicken from the pot, reduce the heat to medium, and add the onions, mushrooms, zucchini, celery, and carrots. Cook, stirring, until the mushrooms begin to brown, about 7 minutes. Add the tomatoes, tomato paste, garlic, wine, and rosemary. Return the chicken to the pot, cover, and simmer until tender, about 1 hour.

MAKES 6 SERVINGS

210 calories per serving, 19 g protein, 7 g fat (1.5 sat), 15 g carbohydrate, 67 mg sodium, 882 mg potassium, 4 g dietary fiber

Exchanges: 3 Vegetable, 2 Lean Meat

CHICKEN CASSOULET

Chicken and beans are flavored with a small amount of sausage in this easy version of a classic dish. But this lighter cassoulet contains just a fraction of the calories and saturated fat that you'd would find in a French country kitchen.

1 tablespoon olive oil
1 pound skinless, boneless chicken breasts
2 large yellow onions, chopped
2 ounces hot Italian turkey sausage
3 medium carrots, cut into chunks
2 celery ribs, chopped
2 cloves garlic, minced
8 sun-dried tomatoes, cut into strips
1 (15½-ounce) can great Northern beans, rinsed and drained
1½ cups low-sodium chicken broth, defatted
1 cup dry white wine
1 teaspoon dried thyme
1 bay leaf

1. Preheat the oven to 350° F.

2. Heat the olive oil in a large Dutch oven over medium heat; add the chicken, onions, and sausage, and cook until the chicken and sausage are brown on both sides. Break up the sausage into small pieces. Add the remaining ingredients; bring to a boil.

3. Bake, covered, for 1 hour. Remove bay leaf before serving.

MAKES 6 SERVINGS

290 calories per serving, 26 g protein, 7 g fat (1 sat), 25 g carbohydrate, 205 mg sodium, 746 mg potassium, 6 g dietary fiber

Exchanges: 4 Vegetable, 2½ Lean Meat, 1 Fat

TURKEY MARSALA

Marsala wine is an inexpensive fortified wine that turns into a wonderful sauce for tender turkey cutlets.

¼ cup all-purpose flour
1 pound thinly sliced turkey cutlets
1 tablespoon olive oil
10 ounces mushrooms, sliced
¾ cup marsala
⅛ teaspoon ground nutmeg
Salt and freshly ground black pepper to taste
2 tablespoons chopped fresh parsley

1. Place the flour in a plastic bag; add the turkey, seal, and shake to lightly coat with flour.

2. Heat the oil in a large heavy skillet over medium heat; cook the turkey until light golden brown on both sides, about 2 minutes on a side. Remove from the skillet and keep warm.

3. Add the mushrooms to the same skillet, and cook, stirring, until softened, about 3 minutes; add the marsala and nutmeg, and cook until the sauce begins to thicken, about 3 minutes.

4. Return the turkey to the skillet, reduce the heat to low, and cook about 4 minutes. Arrange the cutlets and sauce on a platter, season with salt and pepper, and sprinkle with parsley.

MAKES 4 SERVINGS

240 calories per serving, 27 g protein, 6 g fat (1.4 sat), 7 g carbohydrate, 60 mg sodium, 536 mg potassium, 1 g dietary fiber

Exchanges: 1 Vegetable, 3 Lean Meat, 1 Fat

TURKEY TETRAZZINI

I often roast a turkey breast for Sunday dinner and then use the leftovers during the week for sandwiches and for this lower-calorie version of a delicious pasta dish named after a famous Italian opera singer.

6 ounces fettuccine or linguine

3 tablespoons slivered blanched almonds

1 tablespoon olive oil

10 ounces mushrooms, sliced

2 tablespoons all-purpose flour

1 cup skim milk

1¼ cups low-sodium chicken broth, defatted

⅛ teaspoon ground nutmeg

2 cups shredded cooked turkey

1. Cook the pasta according to the package directions.

2. Meanwhile, toast the slivered almonds in a dry skillet over medium-high heat, about 4 minutes, until fragrant and lightly browned; set aside.

3. Heat the olive oil in a large heavy skillet over medium heat, and cook the mushrooms, stirring, for about 3 minutes while sprinkling them with the flour to make a roux (paste).

4. Reduce the heat to low. Add the milk, broth, and nutmeg; cook, stirring, until the sauce begins to thicken. Add the turkey, and cook until heated thoroughly, about 5 minutes.

5. Drain the pasta, and arrange it on a platter. Top with the turkey and sauce. Sprinkle on the toasted almonds and serve immediately.

MAKES 4 SERVINGS

390 calories per serving, 32 g protein, 10 g fat (1.7 sat), 43 g carbohydrate, 300 mg sodium, 690 mg potassium, 2 g dietary fiber

Exchanges: 3 Starch, 2 Lean Meat, I Fat

CHICKEN PARMESAN

To make this easy stove-top chicken Parmesan even quicker, you can use 2 cups of ready-made tomato sauce.

- ¼ cup flour
- 1 pound skinless, boneless chicken breasts
- 1½ tablespoons olive oil
- 1 recipe Easy Tomato Sauce (page 164)
- ¼ cup freshly grated Parmesan cheese

1. Put the flour in a plastic bag, add the chicken, seal, and shake to lightly coat with flour.

2. Heat the olive oil in a large skillet with a cover or in a Dutch oven over medium heat. Cook the chicken until it is lightly browned, about 4 minutes per side.

3. Add the Easy Tomato Sauce, reduce the heat to low, cover, and simmer for 30 minutes, turning the chicken halfway through the cooking time.

4. Sprinkle the chicken with the Parmesan, cover, and cook until the cheese melts, about 5 minutes.

MAKES 4 SERVINGS

310 calories per serving, 33 g protein, 10 g fat (2.8 sat), 23 g carbohydrate, 217 mg sodium, 1,061 mg potassium, 5 g dietary fiber

Exchanges: 4 Vegetable, 3 Lean Meat, 1 Fat

SHRIMP AND ARTICHOKES WITH LEMONY PASTA

This dish is fancy enough for company, but prepared artichokes and precooked shrimp make it extremely fast and easy.

1 lemon

½ pound linguine

1 tablespoon olive oil

½ pound frozen cooked medium shrimp, thawed

2 cloves garlic, minced

1 cup low-sodium chicken broth, defatted

1 cup canned artichoke hearts, drained and quartered

Chopped fresh parsley

1. Wash the lemon and dry it. Make lemon zest by grating the yellow outside peel with the fine side of a cheese grater. Cut the lemon in half and squeeze the juice into a small cup.

2. Cook the pasta according to the package directions; drain and toss with the lemon juice and lemon zest.

3. Heat the olive oil in a large skillet over medium heat; add the shrimp and cook about 1 minute. Then add the garlic, and cook until it is fragrant, about 1 minute. Add the broth and artichokes, and simmer for 5 minutes to heat through. Toss with the pasta and parsley and serve immediately.

MAKES 4 SERVINGS

320 calories per serving, 20 g protein, 5 g fat (0.8 sat), 48 g carbohydrate, 40 mg sodium, 440 mg potassium, 3 g dietary fiber

Exchanges: 3 Starch, 2 Lean Meat

SHRIMP AND PEPPER RISOTTO

This is an elegant shrimp dish that is easy to make. The hot peppers make a nice contrast to the creamy rice.

1 recipe Basic Risotto (page 159)

1 tablespoon olive oil

2 jalapeño peppers, cut into thin strips

1 large red bell pepper, seeded and chopped

½ pound frozen cooked medium shrimp, thawed

1. Prepare the risotto and keep warm.

2. Heat the olive oil in a nonstick skillet over medium heat; add the jalapeño and red bell peppers and cook until they begin to soften, about 2 minutes. Add the shrimp and heat until cooked through, about 3 minutes.

3. Add the peppers and shrimp to the risotto and serve.

MAKES 4 SERVINGS

300 calories per serving, 17 g protein, 7 g fat (0.6 sat), 42 g carbohydrate, 403 mg sodium, 218 mg potassium, 1 g dietary fiber

Exchanges: 2½ Starch, 2 Very Lean Meat, 1 Fat

SIMPLE SALMON

Although restaurant chefs and cookbook authors seem compelled to smother salmon with every imaginable ingredient, fresh salmon is so good it really doesn't need very much embellishment.

1 pound fresh salmon fillet

1 lime, halved

1 teaspoon olive oil

2 tablespoons plain dried bread crumbs

1. Preheat the broiler. Check the salmon for bones; even though it's not a terribly bony fish, any that are there will be firmly embedded.

2. Place the salmon skin side down in a broiler pan. Squeeze one half of the lime over the fish, brush it with the oil, and sprinkle with the bread crumbs.

3. Broil the salmon, without turning, about 6 inches from heat, for 7 to 10 minutes. The fish is done when the flesh is opaque in the center. Cut the remaining lime half into wedges and serve with the salmon.

190 calories, 23 g protein, 9 g fat (1.3 sat), 4 g carbohydrate, 73 mg sodium, 578 mg potassium, 0 g dietary fiber

Exchanges: 3 Lean Meat

CRAB CAKES

....

Crabmeat is expensive so we save it for special occasions. My birthday meal is usually crab cakes, Winter Slaw (page 133), Roasted Potato Sticks (page 137), and Pumpkin Walnut Cheesecake (page 211).

> Olive oil cooking spray
>
> 2 large egg whites
>
> 1 pound lump crabmeat, picked over for cartilage and shells and patted dry
>
> 3 tablespoons reduced-fat mayonnaise
>
> 2 tablespoons freshly squeezed lemon juice
>
> 2 teaspoons Old Bay seasoning
>
> ⅛ teaspoon freshly ground black pepper

1. Preheat the broiler. Spray a baking sheet with cooking spray.

2. Lightly beat the egg whites in a large bowl. Add remaining ingredients, and toss lightly with a fork.

3. Form the crab mixture into 4 patties, and place them in the prepared pan. Lightly spray each patty with cooking spray.

4. Broil the crab cakes until lightly browned, about 5 minutes. Turn and broil 4 to 5 minutes longer. Serve immediately.

MAKES 4 SERVINGS

155 calories per serving, 24 g protein, 5 g fat (0.2 sat), 2 g carbohydrate, 1,243 mg sodium, 331 mg potassium, 0 g dietary fiber

Exchanges: 3 Lean Meat

MEDITERRANEAN FISH BAKE

The key to the wonderful flavor of this dish is sautéing the vegetables before baking.

1 tablespoon olive oil

1 large yellow onion, sliced

1 small zucchini, cut into sticks

1 clove garlic, minced

2 plum tomatoes, chopped

1 roasted red pepper (from a jar), chopped

1 tablespoon capers

2 tablespoons chopped black olives

1 (14-ounce) package frozen haddock, defrosted

¼ cup feta cheese, crumbled

1. Preheat oven to 400° F.

2. Heat the olive oil in a large heavy skillet over medium-low heat. Add the onion, and cook until it begins to soften, about 5 minutes. Add the zucchini and cook until softened, about 5 minutes.

3. Add the garlic, cook for 1 minute. Stir in the tomatoes, red pepper, capers, and olives. Turn off the heat.

4. Place the haddock in a medium casserole dish. Spoon the vegetable mixture on top, and sprinkle with the cheese. Bake until the fish turns opaque and flakes easily with a fork, about 25 minutes.

MAKES 4 SERVINGS

180 calories per serving, 22 g protein, 7 g fat (1.8 sat), 9 g carbohydrate, 356 mg sodium, 630 mg potassium, 2 g dietary fiber

Exchanges: 1 Vegetable, 3 Very Lean Meat, 1 Fat

SIMPLE SOLE

There's no need to serve filets swimming in butter when a little olive oil, lemon juice, and a bit of Parmesan cheese make them taste even better.

1 tablespoon olive oil

1 pound sole fillets

2 tablespoons frozen lemon juice, thawed, or freshly squeezed

2 tablespoons freshly grated Parmesan cheese

1. Preheat the oven to 450° F. Coat the bottom of a baking dish with the olive oil. Add the filets, and turn to coat both sides with the oil. Drizzle the lemon juice on top. Sprinkle the cheese evenly over the fish.

2. Bake until the fish turns opaque and flakes easily with a fork, about 12 minutes.

MAKES 4 SERVINGS

160 calories per serving, 23 g protein, 7 g fat (2 sat), 1 g carbohydrate, 206 mg sodium, 308 mg potassium, 0 g dietary fiber

Exchanges: 3 Very Lean Meat, 1 Fat

MEDITERRANEAN TUNA SALAD

Serve this tuna salad on a bed of greens with some sliced fresh tomato.

1 tablespoon olive oil

½ teaspoon dried thyme

1 tablespoon frozen lemon juice, thawed, or freshly squeezed

1 (6½-ounce) can water-packed albacore tuna, drained

1 (15½-ounce) can great Northern beans, drained and rinsed

1 bunch watercress

Salt and freshly ground black pepper to taste

1. Whisk the olive oil, thyme, and lemon juice together in a small bowl.

2. Toss the tuna, beans, and watercress together in a serving bowl. Add the dressing, and toss to mix. Season with salt and pepper. Chill in the refrigerator for 1 hour before serving.

MAKES 4 SERVINGS

220 calories per serving, 21 g protein, 5 g fat (0.7 sat) 23 g carbohydrate, 190 mg sodium, 600 mg potassium, 6 g dietary fiber

Exchanges: 1 Starch, 1 Vegetable, 2 Very Lean Meat, 1 Fat

♥

CHAPTER 17

Small Meals and Snacks

The recipes in this chapter are designed for people on the go. Included are two quick-and-easy breakfast recipes, ideas for brown-bag lunches, and a variety of snacks. The emphasis is on take-along food that is good for you, which just may help you from becoming so hungry that you lunge at the next glazed doughnut you happen by.

To snack or not to snack is a decision we all have to make, and there are certainly pluses and minuses for three squares versus five small meals a day. Three meals without snacks makes the most sense for those whose appetite is triggered to make them overeat each time they sit down to eat. If you have this problem, fewer eating episodes throughout the day may be a better way to go. Yet others may find that having a small snack helps ward off hunger and avoid becoming so ravenous that they overeat at the next meal. Another plus is that smaller meals present the body with less of a glucose challenge at any given time, which makes it easier for insulin to do its job in the face of insulin resistance.

Whether you decide to eat more or less at one time, I hope the recipes here will help you stick with the right stuff, and not even give that glazed doughnut a second thought.

BREAKFAST CAKES

Although these are similar to muffins, I call them Breakfast Cakes, because they are intended to stand in as a great high-fiber breakfast. They are also rich in vitamins, minerals, and omega-3s from the walnuts, flaxseeds, and canola oil.

    Canola oil cooking spray
    1 tablespoon flaxseeds
    ½ cup walnut halves
    1 cup oat bran cereal
    1 cup quick-cooking oats
    1 cup Bran Buds cereal
    ¼ cup firmly packed brown sugar
    1 teaspoon ground cinnamon
    ¼ teaspoon salt
    1 orange
    1¼ cups buttermilk
    1 large egg
    ¼ cup canola oil
    ½ cup chopped dried apricots
    2 teaspoons granulated sugar

1. Preheat the oven to 350° F. Spray a heavy baking sheet with cooking spray and spread the flaxseeds and walnuts on the sheet. Toast them in the oven for 7 minutes, cool, and coarsly chop.

2. Meanwhile, mix the oat bran, oats, Bran Buds cereal, brown sugar, cinnamon, and salt in a large bowl.

3. Wash the orange and dry it. Make 1 teaspoon of orange zest by grating the orange peel with the fine side of a cheese grater. Measure the buttermilk in a large glass measuring cup; add the orange zest, egg, and canola oil. Beat the wet ingredients with a fork, add to the dry ingredients, and mix until moistened.

4. Fold the flaxseeds, walnuts, and apricots into the batter. Scoop up the batter with a ¼-cup measuring cup, and drop onto the baking sheet. Press each mound of batter into a cake about 1 inch thick, and sprinkle the tops of each cake with a small amount of granulated sugar. Bake until a toothpick inserted in the center comes out clean, 25 to 30 minutes.

MAKES 12 CAKES

185 calories per cake, 6 g protein, 8 g fat (0.8 sat), 23 g carbohydrate, 123 mg sodium, 315 mg potassium, 4 g dietary fiber

Exchanges: 1½ Starch, 2 Fat

Variations

♥ Lemon zest can be substituted for the orange zest.

♥ I use dried apricots because they have a low glycemic index and they're rich in carotenoids; but if you really don't like apricots, substitute ¼ cup currants.

TIP

Make these on the weekend for quick breakfasts during the busy week. If they are to be eaten within 2 days, they keep well in a tin. For longer storage, wrap them individually and freeze.

PEACH ALMOND SMOOTHIE

You need a well-stocked healthful pantry for this recipe, but each ingredient contributes to this nutrition-packed breakfast in a glass: peaches for carotenoids and fiber; oat bran for more fiber; milk and yogurt for calcium, potassium, and friendly bacteria; egg white powder for protein; and canola oil for richness, monos, and omega-3s.

1 cup skim milk

1 cup nonfat vanilla yogurt

1 cup frozen sliced peaches

2 tablespoons oat bran

2 tablespoons powdered egg whites

1 tablespoon canola oil

2 drops pure almond extract

Add all the ingredients to a blender. Blend until smooth. Divide between two glasses and serve.

MAKES 2 SERVINGS

290 calories per serving, 21 g protein, 8 g fat (0.7 sat), 36 g carbohydrate, 185 mg sodium, 654 mg potassium, 3 g dietary fiber

Exchanges: I Fat-Free Milk, I Fruit, I Starch, I Very Lean Meat, I Fat

Variations

♥   One cup fresh sliced peaches may be substituted for the frozen; ¼ cup canned light peaches may also be used.

♥   Substitute flaxseed oil (page 101) for some or all of the canola oil, if you want to boost your omega-3s further.

TIP

Be careful with the pure almond extract—any more than one or two drops is overpowering.

PEANUTTY HUMMUS

If you eat as much hummus as we do, it is well worth it to make your own because it is so easy. It is also very inexpensive if you use peanut butter in place of tahini (sesame paste), which is used in traditional recipes. The flavor is just slightly peanutty, and, I think, just as good.

1 (15½-ounce) can chickpeas, drained and rinsed

¼ cup frozen lemon juice, thawed, or freshly squeezed

2 tablespoons smooth natural peanut butter

1 tablespoon olive oil

1 garlic clove, finely minced

Place all the ingredients in a blender or food processor. (If you're using a blender, put the lemon juice in first.) Blend until smooth.

MAKES 1½ CUPS

124 calories per ¼ cup, 5 g protein, 6 g fat (0.8 sat), 14 g carbohydrate, 307 mg sodium, 188 mg potassium, 4 g dietary fiber

Exchanges: 1½ Starch, I Very Lean Meat, I Fat

Variations

𝒱 Make your own gourmet hummus by adding any of the following: cracked black pepper, roasted red peppers, chopped black olives, green onions, or lemon zest to make it *really* lemony.

TIP
One or more roasted garlic cloves can be substituted for the fresh.

ROASTED RED PEPPER SPREAD

....

Roasted red peppers are commonly used in sauces and spreads throughout the Mediterranean. Using roasted red peppers from a jar makes this simple dish a snap. Spread it on Crostini (page 191), use it as a vegetable dip, or serve it alongside chicken or fish.

1 small clove garlic, peeled

⅛ teaspoon salt

1 (12-ounce) jar roasted red peppers, drained

½ cup walnuts

Pinch cayenne pepper

1. Cut the garlic clove in half; if there is a green sprout in the center, remove it. Mash the garlic with the salt. (This tempers the raw garlic taste.)

2. Place the roasted peppers in a food processor or blender. Add the garlic, walnuts, and cayenne pepper, and process until creamy.

MAKES 1½ CUPS

75 calories per ¼ cup, 2 g protein, 6 g fat (0.09 sat), 4 g carbohydrate, 46 mg sodium, 120 mg potassium, 1 g dietary fiber

Exchanges: I Vegetable, I Fat

TIP
Jarred roasted red peppers are usually near the olives or with the Italian specialty foods in the supermarket.

CROSTINI

Serve crostini instead of packaged crackers made with hydrogenated oil. They're dry and crisp and just right for smearing with healthy spreads.

> 1 (16-inch-long) loaf French bread (baguette)

Preheat the oven to 350° F. Slice the bread into ¼-inch-thick slices and spread evenly on a baking sheet. Bake for 20 minutes, or until dry and golden. Cool, and store wrapped in aluminum foil or in a covered tin if not using immediately.

MAKES 64 CROSTINI

20 calories each, 1 g protein, 4 g carbohydrate, 0 g fat, 22 mg sodium, 8 mg potassium, 0 g dietary fiber

Exchanges: ¼ starch

YOGURT-MUSTARD DIP

Full-fat yogurt makes this dip rich and creamy, yet there's no need to worry about getting too much saturated fat, because as a vegetable dip, it is eaten in small amounts and not by the cup.

> 1 cup full-fat plain yogurt
> 3 tablespoons coarse-grained brown mustard
> Pinch sweetener (optional)

Mix the yogurt and mustard together in a small bowl. Taste, and add a bit of sugar or sugar substitute if it's too tangy. Refrigerated, this dip will keep for 2 days.

MAKES 1¼ CUPS

28 calories per ¼ cup, 2 g protein, 2 g fat (0.9 sat), 2 g carbohydrate, 28 mg sodium, 71 mg potassium, 0 g dietary fiber

Exchanges: ¼ Milk

ROASTED EGGPLANT AND GARLIC SPREAD

Spread this flavorful dip on Crostini (page 191) for a tasty, healthy appetizer.

Olive or canola oil cooking spray
2 small eggplants
1 small head garlic
12 stuffed green olives
1 tablespoon olive oil

1. Preheat the oven to 350° F. Spray a heavy baking sheet with cooking spray. Pierce the eggplants in four or five places with a fork; place in the baking sheet.

2. Prepare the garlic according to the Roasted Garlic recipe (page 136), and place it in the baking sheet with the eggplants. Bake until the eggplants are tender, about 40 minutes.

3. Cut the eggplants in half and scoop the pulp into a medium bowl; discard the skins. Separate the garlic cloves and squeeze the roasted garlic into the eggplant.

4. Slice the olives into thin rounds; add to the eggplant along with the olive oil. Mix the ingredients together with a fork. Refrigerated, this spread keeps for 3 days.

MAKES 2 CUPS

30 calories per ¼ cup, 1 g protein, 3 g fat (0.3 sat), 2 g carbohydrate, 122 mg sodium, 68 mg potassium, 1 g dietary fiber

Exchanges: 1 Fat

PITA CRISPS

....

Pita crisps are great with Roasted Red Pepper Spread (page 190) or hummus. Use 6-inch whole wheat pita breads that are sold in the bread aisle of most supermarkets.

>   3 whole wheat pita breads

Preheat the oven to 400° F. Cut each pita into eighths, as you would cut a pizza; then separate each triangle at the fold. (Each pita makes 16 triangles.) Arrange the triangles on a baking sheet and bake until crisp, about 10 minutes. Stored in a tin, the pita crisps will keep for 1 week.

MAKES 48 CHIPS

4 calories per chip, 0 g protein, 0 g fat, 1 g carbohydrate, 2 mg sodium, 1 mg potassium, 0 g dietary fiber

Exchanges: 1 Starch for 15 pita crisps

EASY GARLIC BREAD

....

Try to find a bread that is made with half whole wheat flour, which makes it chewier and higher in fiber than bread made from white flour alone.

>   1 clove garlic
>   4 teaspoons olive oil
>   8 slices crusty Italian bread

1. Preheat the oven to 350° F.

2. Peel the garlic and either press in a garlic press or mince very finely. In a small bowl, combine the garlic with the olive oil.

3. Brush each slice of the bread with the oil mixture, place in a baking sheet, and warm for about 10 minutes.

MAKES 8 SLICES

105 calories per slice, 3 g protein, 2 g fat (0.3 sat), 17 g carbohydrate, 150 mg sodium, 25 mg potassium, 1 g dietary fiber

Exchanges: 1 Starch, ½ Fat

NOTE: It is unsafe to make extra garlic and oil to store for future use, because of the risk of botulism. Make only as much as you need, and use it right away.

MEDITERRANEAN POCKET

....

If you're tired of turkey and tuna for lunch, this flavorful vegetarian sandwich will be a welcome change.

> 3 strips roasted red peppers from a jar, chopped
> 2 tablespoons chopped olives
> 1 ounce feta cheese, crumbled
> Pinch of dried oregano
> ½ cup chopped Romaine lettuce
> 2 teaspoons Basic Dressing (page 132)
> 1 (6-inch) whole wheat pita pocket

1. In a small bowl, toss peppers, olives, feta, oregano, and chopped lettuce with the Basic Dressing.

2. Slice the pita in half and spoon in the filling.

MAKES 1 SANDWICH

120 calories per sandwich, 5 g protein, 6 g fat (2.5 sat), 13 g carbohydrate, 290 mg sodium, 158 mg potassium, 3 g dietary fiber

Exchanges: 1 Vegetable, ½ Starch, 1 Medium-Fat Meat

PARMESAN CRISPS

Cayenne pepper enhances the cheese flavor of these homemade crackers, which are good with soup.

2 cups quick-cooking oats

¼ cup freshly grated Parmesan cheese

¼ teaspoon cayenne pepper

⅛ teaspoon salt

1 large egg

1 large egg white

2 tablespoons canola oil

1. Preheat the oven to 400° F. Place the oats in a blender or food proccessor and grind until they have the consistency of flour.

2. Mix the oat flour, Parmesan, cayenne pepper, and salt in a medium bowl.

3. Beat the egg, egg white, and canola oil in a separate bowl; add to the dry ingredients, and stir until moistened.

4. Place the dough by the rounded tablespoonful in a baking sheet. Press into 20 thin round cakes, about 2½ inches across.

5. Bake 10 minutes, until golden. Cool and store in a covered tin.

MAKES 20 CRACKERS

55 calories per cracker, 2 g protein, 2 g fat (0.6 sat), 5 g carbohydrate, 43 mg sodium, 36 mg potassium, 1 g dietary fiber

Exchanges: ½ **Starch,** ½ **Fat**

YOGURT CHEESE

Creamy Yogurt Cheese is a healthy alternative to cream cheese and sour cream, because it contains more calcium and much less fat. Buy the best, sweetest-tasting plain yogurt you can find (page 106). Also, make sure the yogurt does not contain guar gum or other thickeners, as they will prevent the liquid from draining out.

> 2 cups plain nonfat yogurt

Place a fine-mesh colander over a medium bowl. Spoon the yogurt into the colander, and let it drain. Cover with plastic wrap, and store in the refrigerator for at least 4 hours to make a stiff yogurt cheese. (It is ready when the bowl contains a good amount of liquid and the yogurt has thickened to the consistency of cream cheese.)

MAKES 1 CUP

64 calories per ¼ cup, 7 g protein, 0 g fat, 9 g carbohydrate, 87 mg sodium, 290 mg potassium, 0 g dietary fiber

Exchanges: 1 Fat-Free Milk

YOGURT CHEESE SPREAD

Adding a little good fat to Yogurt Cheese makes it rich without raising your cholesterol. Here's where you will notice the flavor of quality olive oil.

> 1 tablespoon olive oil, preferably extra-virgin
> 2 green onions, chopped
> 3 tablespoons red bell pepper, chopped
> 1 cup Yogurt Cheese (above)

Stir the olive oil, green onions, and pepper into the yogurt cheese.

MAKES ABOUT 1 CUP

45 calories per ¼ cup, 3 g protein, 2 grams fat (0.04 sat), 5 g carbohydrate, 77 mg sodium, 149 mg potassium, 0 g dietary fiber

Exchanges: ½ Reduced-Fat Milk

Variations

❤ Substitute chopped fresh cayenne or jalapeño pepper for the sweet pepper for little hot bits of flavor.

VEGETABLE NACHOS

....

A far cry from the greasy nachos you get in a restaurant, these nachos taste a whole lot better and are a whole lot better for you. Use baked, rather than fried, chips.

Olive or canola oil cooking spray
24 large whole baked tortilla chips
½ cup prepared black bean dip
¾ cup prepared thick salsa
½ cup shredded low-fat Cheddar cheese
¼ cup chopped green or red bell pepper
1 green onion, thinly sliced

1. Preheat the oven to 350° F. Coat a baking sheet or jelly roll pan with a thin layer of cooking spray.

2. Spread the tortilla chips in the baking sheet. Spoon a small amount of the bean dip and the salsa on each chip, sprinkle with the cheese, and top with the pepper and onion.

3. Bake until the cheese is melted, about 10 minutes.

MAKES 4 SERVINGS

130 calories per serving, 8 g protein, 4 g fat (0.3 sat), 17 g carbohydrate, 253 mg sodium, 218 mg potassium, 2 g dietary fiber

Exchanges: 1 Starch, 1 Lean Meat

Variations

𝒱 Yellow or white onions may be substituted for green.

𝒱 Plain canned black beans can be mashed with a fork and substituted for the black bean dip.

TIPS

Thin salsa makes soggy nachos, so be sure to buy thick salsa or drain thin salsa before using. Black bean dip is usually found in the Mexican food section of the supermarket.

CHIVEY CHEESE SPREAD

I can never find ready-made low-fat cottage cheese with chives, so I make my own and add chopped red bell pepper and ground black pepper to make it really good. This spread is great on rye crackers.

> 2 tablespoons chopped chives, fresh or dried
>
> 2 tablespoons finely chopped red bell pepper
>
> 1 cup low-fat cottage cheese
>
> Freshly ground black pepper to taste

Mix the chives, bell pepper, and black pepper with the cottage cheese in a small bowl with a lid. Store refrigerated for up to 2 days.

MAKES 1 CUP

50 calories per ¼ cup, 8 g protein, 1 g fat (0.6 sat), 2 g carbohydrate, 230 mg sodium, 57 mg potassium, 0 g dietary fiber

Exchanges: 1 Lean Meat

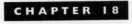

CHAPTER 18

Treat Yourself

My philosophy about desserts is to make them work with your diet, and not against it. For example, we're supposed to be eating more fruits anyway, so it makes sense to make them really yummy by sprinkling them with bits of flavor boosters and baking them in the oven. Dairy products for calcium? Yogurt Cheese and Yogurt Cream are just about the best sources of calcium you can come up with, and nothing goes better with cooked fruit desserts. And now that we know how healthy oats and nuts are, there's really no limit to the possibilities.

In this chapter, I've given you just a sampling of what you can do with these wholesome ingredients. When you go to the trouble of making a dessert from scratch, make sure you get something for those calories. And it's really not that hard once you get going and realize that the old desserts consisting almost exclusively of sugar, fat, and white flour simply do not satisfy as well as desserts made with just a little sugar, fruit, nuts, whole grains, and low-fat dairy products. Again, making sure that what you eat contains fiber is key for feeling satiated, not to mention how it slows the postmeal rise in blood sugar.

Just to set the record straight, I really have nothing against artificial sweeteners. I do, however, worry that they help foster the idea that sugar is the problem in type 2 diabetes: "If I use sugar replacers, I will be okay."

But sugar should be near the bottom of the list of concerns, after calories, exercise, type of fat, and getting enough fiber, fruits, vegetables, whole grains, and low-fat dairy products. I use small amounts of sugar in my recipes to show you how you can make a little go a long way.

Back in 1994, the American Diabetes Association (ADA) explained that gram for gram, sugar (simple carbohydrates) has the same effect on blood sugar as starch (complex carbohydrates). This information has been very slow to catch on. Nonetheless, the ADA's stand is that using reasonable amounts of white table sugar (sucrose) and other simple carbohydrates as part of a meal does not impair blood sugar control in either type 1 or type 2 diabetes.

FIVE TRICKS FOR MAKING DESSERTS TASTE SWEETER

- Use extra vanilla—it enhances sweetness.

- Use calorie-free natural flavors like lemon zest, orange zest, pure almond extract, cinnamon, nutmeg, and ginger.

- Use flavorful fortified wines, such as Madeira, marsala, and port; most of the alcohol calories will cook off, leaving a wonderful flavor behind.

- Rely on the natural sweetness in fruits, which becomes more intense when fruits are cooked.

- Sprinkle a little granulated sugar on the outside of baked goods, such as muffins; the sugar will caramelize in the oven and form a sweet, crispy crust that hits your mouth immediately.

PEARS BAKED IN MADEIRA

When cooked this way, pears take on a creamy texture and become intensely sweet; the Yogurt Cream tastes pleasantly tart in comparison.

> 2 pears
>
> 4 teaspoons Madeira wine
>
> 1 cup Yogurt Cream (page 202)

1. Preheat the oven to 400° F. Cut the pears in half, remove the cores, and place them cut side up in a small baking dish.

2. Spoon 1 teaspoon Madeira over each pear half. Bake for 30 minutes, until the pears are soft and creamy.

3. Serve each pear half with ¼ cup Yogurt Cream.

MAKES 4 SERVINGS

135 calories per serving, 6 g protein, 2 g fat (1.1 sat), 23 g carbohydrate, 80 mg sodium, 353 mg potassium, 2 g dietary fiber

Exchanges: I Fruit, I Fat-Free Milk

Variation

♥ If you're serving guests, you can garnish the Yogurt Cream with a crushed gingersnap cookie; one crushed cookie adds 15 calories and 3 grams carbohydrate per serving.

YOGURT CREAM

Yogurt Cream is made the same way as Yogurt Cheese, but with a shorter draining time. Be careful with pure almond extract: It's so concentrated that more than a drop or two is overpowering.

> 2 cups plain nonfat yogurt
> 4 teaspoons sugar
> 1 teaspoon pure vanilla extract
> 1 drop pure almond extract

1. Place a cheesecloth or a large coffee filter in a colander. Set the colander over a bowl.

2. Add the yogurt, cover with plastic wrap, and place it in the refrigerator. Allow the yogurt to drain until it is thick but still creamy, about 1 hour.

3. Transfer the yogurt cream to a bowl; stir in the sugar, vanilla, and almond extract.

MAKES 4 SERVINGS

75 calories per serving, 6 g protein, 0 g fat, 12 g carbohydrate, 90 mg sodium, 289 mg potassium, 0 g fiber

Exchanges: I Fat-Free Milk

CINNAMON SCIENCE

If you're wondering why most of the dessert recipes in this book call for cinnamon, there is a very good reason. Besides its wonderful taste and smell, cinnamon has been shown to enhance insulin sensitivity. U.S. Department of Agriculture (USDA) researcher Richard Anderson, who led the chromium study discussed on page 81, measured the ability of thirty-one foods and twenty-two spices to potentiate insulin's action in live cells. Cinnamon, cloves, turmeric, bay leaves, and apple pie spice were the most effective spices, each of which tripled insulin's effect. After the study was released, the USDA research center received calls from people reporting improvements in blood sugar from adding ¼ teaspoon ground cinnamon (or less) to foods. Of course, using these spices is not as important as exercise and weight control; but even if the effect is small, it's a painless way to give insulin a little boost.

BAKED APPLES WITH CRUNCHY TOPPING

These are like individual apple crisps, but require less work.

2 apples
2 tablespoons frozen lemon juice, thawed, or freshly squeezed
2 tablespoons quick-cooking or regular oats
2 teaspoons firmly packed brown sugar
½ teaspoon ground cinnamon
Pinch salt
2 teaspoons walnut or canola oil

1. Preheat the oven to 350° F. Cut the apples in half and remove the cores. Spoon 1 tablespoon of the lemon juice over the cut side of the apples.

2. Toss the oats, sugar, cinnamon, and salt together in a small bowl.

3. Stir in the oil and the remaining 1 tablespoon of lemon juice. Spoon the oat mixture into the hollow in the center of each apple half. Bake until the topping is crisp, about 45 minutes.

MAKES 4 SERVINGS

80 calories per serving, 1 g protein, 3 g fat (0.4 sat), 15 g carbohydrate, 68 mg sodium, 107 mg potassium, 2 g fiber

Exchanges: 1 Fruit, ½ Fat

ALL-SEASON FRUIT SALAD

There's nothing like a fresh fruit salad in season, but with this combination of fresh, frozen, and canned fruit you can have the taste of summer any time of the year.

1 banana, peeled and sliced
1 cup frozen mixed berries
1 (7¾-ounce) can light peaches, drained
2 oranges

1. Combine the banana, berries, and peaches in a medium bowl.

2. Quarter the oranges, remove the skins, and cut each quarter into bite-sized pieces.

3. Add the oranges to the other fruit. Refrigerate until the berries are thawed, about 1 hour.

MAKES 4 SERVINGS

95 calories per serving, 1 g protein, 0.4 g fat (0.07 sat), 24 g carbohydrate, 2 mg sodium, 316 mg potassium, 4 g dietary fiber

Exchanges: 1½ Fruit

Variations

𝒱 Use fresh berries and peaches when available.

𝒱 Add or substitute other fruits, such as kiwis, apples, grapes, mangoes, pears, or melon balls. The calorie and fiber counts per cup of fruit salad will be similar to those given.

PLUM TART

My friend Patsy Jamieson introduced me to the flavor of cooked plums when she brought a fabulous plum tart to one of our first *Eating Well* magazine parties. This plum filling is much like Patsy's, but I use an oatmeal crust to make a true fruit 'n' fiber dessert.

FOR THE CRUST

1 cup quick-cooking oats

¼ cup whole wheat flour

2 teaspoons firmly packed brown sugar

1 large egg white

2 tablespoons canola oil

⅛ teaspoon salt

FOR THE FILLING

8 large ripe plums

3 tablespoons frozen lemon juice, thawed, or freshly squeezed

¼ cup firmly packed brown sugar

2 teaspoons ground cinnamon

1 tablespoon all-purpose flour

1. Make the crust. Preheat the oven to 350° F. Place the oats in a blender or food processor, and process until they resemble a flour.

2. Place the oats, flour, salt, and brown sugar in the center of a 9-inch pie plate; toss with a fork. Make a well in the center of the flour mixture, add the egg white and oil; mix thoroughly. Pat the crust to cover the bottom and the sides of the pie plate. Bake the shell for 10 minutes.

3. Make the filling. Thinly slice the unpeeled plums, and place them in a large bowl. Toss with the lemon juice, sugar, cinnamon, and flour.

4. Spoon the filling into the partially baked pie crust. Bake for 45 minutes, until the plums are tender.

MAKES 8 SERVINGS

190 calories per serving, 5 g protein, 5 g fat (0.8 sat), 33 g carbohydrate, 75 mg sodium, 230 mg potassium, 5 g dietary fiber

Exchanges: I Fruit, I Starch, I Fat

PEACHES AND CREAM

Plain peaches are transformed into an elegant dessert when you roast them in the oven.

2 large ripe peaches
2 teaspoons firmly packed brown sugar
2 tablespoons freshly squeezed lemon juice
½ teaspoon ground cinnamon
1 cup Yogurt Cream (page 202)

1. Preheat the oven to 400° F.

2. Wash the peaches well to remove the fuzz from the skin, but do not remove the skin. Cut the peaches in half and remove the pits.

3. Whisk the sugar with the lemon juice in a small bowl.

4. Arrange the peaches cut side up in a baking dish. Drizzle them with the sugar mixture. Sprinkle each with a bit of the cinnamon.

5. Roast the peaches for 30 to 35 minutes, until tender. Check about halfway through to make sure they're not beginning to burn. If they are, loosen them and add a little water to the bottom of the dish.

6. Serve warm with Yogurt Cream.

MAKES 4 SERVINGS

140 calories per serving, 6 g protein, 2 g fat (0.8 sat), 26 g carbohydrate, 80 mg sodium, 312 mg potassium, 1 g dietary fiber

Exchanges: ½ Fruit, 1 Fat-Free Milk

Variation

♥   Nectarines may be substituted for the peaches.

PECAN CURRANT DROPS

Here, the oats have to be ground into a flour to keep the dough from being too crumbly.

1¾ cup quick-cooking oats

3 tablespoons chopped pecans

¼ cup firmly packed brown sugar

1 teaspoon ground cinnamon

¼ teaspoon salt

1 large egg

1 large egg white

3 tablespoons canola oil

2 teaspoons pure vanilla extract

2 tablespoons currants

1. Preheat oven to 350° F. Place the oats in a blender or food proccessor, and process them until they have the consistency of flour. Spread the pecans in a heavy baking sheet, and bake for 5 minutes to toast them. (Set the timer so they don't burn.)

2. Mix the oat flour, sugar, cinnamon, and salt in a medium bowl. In a small bowl, beat the egg, egg white, canola oil, and vanilla.

3. Add the egg mixture to the dry ingredients, and stir until moistened. Mix in the currants and pecans.

4. Drop the dough by the tablespoonful onto a heavy baking sheet. Bake for 12 minutes, until lightly browned.

MAKES 25 COOKIES

60 calories per cookie, 1 g protein, 3 g fat (0.5 sat), 7 g carbohydrate, 27 mg sodium, 43 mg potassium, 1 g dietary fiber

Exchanges: ½ **Starch, 1 Fat**

PEANUT BUTTER DROPS

Allow plenty of time to preheat the oven—the dough mixes up so quickly that it will be ready before the oven is hot.

1½ cups quick-cooking oats

1 cup crunchy natural peanut butter

¼ cup firmly packed brown sugar

1 egg white

¼ teaspoon salt

1 tablespoon pure vanilla extract

1. Preheat the oven to 350° F.

2. Mix all the ingredients in a medium bowl until creamy.

3. Drop the dough by rounded teaspoonful onto a heavy baking sheet. Bake for 12 minutes, until browned.

MAKES 28 COOKIES

80 calories per cookie, 3 g protein, 5 g fat (0.9 sat), 6 g carbohydrate, 62 mg sodium, 84 mg potassium, 1 g dietary fiber

Exchanges: ½ Starch, 1 Fat

CHOCOLATE HAZELNUT DROPS

These cookies are better for you than most because of the soluble fiber in the oats. Use real semisweet chocolate, because the fat in the cocoa butter does not raise blood cholesterol like the fat in imitation chocolate (not to mention how much better it tastes).

¼ cup chopped hazelnuts

4 ounces semisweet chocolate

1½ cups quick-cooking oats

1 tablespoon sugar

2 teaspoons pure vanilla extract

⅛ teaspoon salt

2 tablespoons brewed coffee

1 large egg

1. Preheat the oven to 350° F. Spread the hazelnuts in a heavy baking sheet and toast in oven for 5 minutes.

2. Meanwhile, melt the chocolate over very low heat in a heavy medium saucepan. Stir and watch carefully so the chocolate doesn't burn; remove the pan from the heat as soon as the chocolate has melted.

3. Leave the melted chocolate in the pan; stir in the oats, sugar, vanilla, salt, and coffee. Beat the egg and fold into the dough. Stir in the toasted hazelnuts.

4. Drop the cookies by the teaspoonful into the baking sheet. Bake for 12 minutes.

MAKES 25 COOKIES

55 calories per cookie, I g protein, 2 g fat (0.2 sat), 7 g carbohydrate, 17 mg sodium, 49 mg potassium, I g dietary fiber

Exchanges: ½ Starch, ½ Fat

STRAWBERRY CHEESE PIE

Aside from being delicious, this pie has a lot going for it: calcium from the yogurt filling, fiber from the crust and strawberries, and a slew of other good things from its wholesome ingredients.

FOR THE CRUST

1 cup quick-cooking oats

¼ cup whole wheat flour

⅛ teaspoon salt

2 teaspoons sugar

1 large egg white

2 tablespoons canola oil

1 orange

2 cups fresh strawberries, hulled

½ cup reduced-sugar strawberry preserves

¼ cup sugar

3 cups stiff Yogurt Cheese (page 196)

1. Preheat the oven to 350° F. Place the oats in a blender or food processor, and process until they resemble a flour.

2. Make the crust. Place the oats, flour, salt, and sugar in the center of a 9-inch pie plate; toss together with a fork. Place the egg white and oil in the center of the flour mixture and mix thoroughly with a fork. Pat the crust into the bottom and up along the sides of the pan. Bake the shell for 20 minutes. Remove from the oven and let cool.

3. Make the filling. Wash and dry the orange, and make 1 teaspoon orange zest by grating the orange skin with the fine side of a cheese grater; set aside. Slice the orange in half and squeeze out 2 teaspoons of juice. Slice the strawberries and mix them in a medium bowl with the orange juice and strawberry preserves.

4. In another bowl, stir the sugar and orange zest into the Yogurt Cheese. Spoon the yogurt mixture into the pie shell and spread the strawberry mixture over top. (If the strawberries are not very juicy, you may need to add a little more orange juice to make the topping spreadable.) Refrigerate the pie until firm, about 2 hours. Serve.

MAKES 8 SERVINGS; I (9-INCH) PIE

245 calories per serving, 13 g protein, 5 g fat (0.8 sat), 39 g carbohydrate, 172 mg sodium, 553 mg potassium, 2 g dietary fiber

Exchanges: I Fruit, I Reduced-Fat Milk, I Starch

PUMPKIN WALNUT CHEESECAKE

This light-as-air cheesecake is my rendition of the delicious, very rich pumpkin cheese-cake served in the fall at one of my favorite Italian restaurants. The "crust" couldn't be easier; it's just chopped walnuts sprinkled on the bottom of the pan.

6 large egg whites

Olive oil or canola oil cooking spray

½ cup walnut halves, chopped

1 tablespoon molasses

1 (15-ounce) container part-skim ricotta cheese

1 (15-ounce) can pumpkin purée

⅓ cup brown sugar, packed

1 tablespoon pure vanilla extract

1½ teaspoons ground cinnamon

½ teaspoon ground nutmeg

1. Preheat the oven to 350° F. In a large bowl, beat the egg whites until soft peaks form.

2. Spray a 9-inch springform pan or deep soufflé dish with cooking spray. Spread the walnuts evenly over the bottom of the pan. Put the pan in the oven for 10 minutes to lightly toast the nuts.

3. In another large bowl, mix together the molasses, ricotta, pumpkin, brown sugar, vanilla, and spices. Fold in the egg whites by gently stirring with a rubber spatula.

4. Remove the pan from the oven. Carefully pour the batter over the walnuts, keeping them spread out as evenly as possible. Bake until a toothpick inserted in the center comes out clean, about 45 minutes. Cool and refrigerate for at least 2 hours before cutting.

MAKES 12 SERVINGS; 1 (9-INCH) CAKE

150 calories per serving, 7 g protein, 6 g fat (2 sat), 19 g carbohydrate, 75 mg sodium, 223 mg potassium, 1 g dietary fiber

Exchanges: 1 Starch, 1 Very Lean Meat, 1 Fat

CRUNCHY BAKED BANANAS

Yogurt Cream is a nice foil to the sweetness of the bananas, which intensifies when you bake them.

Olive or canola oil cooking spray

2 bananas, peeled and sliced in half lengthwise

¼ teaspoon ground cinnamon

2 tablespoons chopped walnuts

1 cup Yogurt Cream (page 202)

1. Preheat the oven to 350° F. Spray a small baking dish with cooking spray.

2. Place the banana halves side by side in the baking dish; spray with cooking spray. Sprinkle them with the cinnamon and then with the chopped walnuts.

3. Bake for 20 minutes; serve with Yogurt Cream.

MAKES 4 SERVINGS

150 calories per serving, 8 g protein, 3 g fat (0.3), 26 g carbohydrate, 88 mg sodium, 536 mg potassium, 1 g dietary fiber

Exchanges: 1 Fruit, 1 Fat-Free Milk

♡

Questions and Answers

Q: Why should I bother making the changes suggested in this book when I can take pills to control my blood sugar?

If you're overweight, don't exercise, and eat a bad diet, taking drugs is really only a Band-Aid approach because you are not working on the underlying problem. But if you are doing what you can to maintain a healthy lifestyle and still need an oral hypoglycemic agent, this is another story. Everyone is different and sometimes a particularly bad set of genes might cause a person to have high blood sugar even when he or she is not overweight, eats well, and exercises every day. The same is true for people who have heart disease or hypertension; sometimes lifestyle changes are simply not enough. The good news is that there are now new drugs that are more effective than ever at working with diet and exercise to overcome insulin resistance.

Q: Is there any reason that a person with type 1 diabetes can't use the recipes in this book?

No. Although the book was written specifically with the priorities for people with type 2 diabetes in mind, the recipes can be used by people with type 1 diabetes because they are based on principles of healthy eating that apply to everyone. In fact, the emphasis on good fats is also ideal for people with type 1 diabetes; however, the meal plans in this book are not recommended for this group because they may be too low in calories or not consistent enough in carbohydrate content from meal to meal to match specific insulin regimens. A registered dietitian or diabetes educator can help create an appropriate meal plan based on the recipes for a person with type 1 diabetes.

Q: What if I have already made diet changes that have helped me, and I don't need detailed meal plans?

By all means, stick with any positive changes you have made. This book gives you examples of healthy ways of eating; however, it is up to you to pick what works for you and incorporate it into your everyday life. For example, if you're like most people, you eat about seven different meals for dinner and repeat them over and over. So if you find you really a like certain new recipe—say, Chicken Cacciatore (page 175) or Turkey Marsala (page 177)—and you start making it instead of picking up fast-food chicken once a week, you will have made a significant improvement to your diet. And if you take the message about vegetables to heart by eating The Big Salad (page 130) on a regular basis, you will not only take a big step toward controlling your weight, blood sugar, and blood pressure but also cut your cancer risk. These types of changes, combined with thirty minutes of exercise each day—the one change that is not optional—go a very long way toward improving the negative health effects of our modern environment.

Q: I have just learned that I have impaired glucose tolerance, and I haven't made any changes yet. Where should I start?

You are very lucky to have caught the problem in this early stage. The first thing to do is start walking every day; see Chapter 4 for advice on how to get started. Then decide how motivated you are about making changes to your diet, whether you want to take things one step at a time, or go all out and make a complete diet overhaul. It would also be a good idea to see a certified diabetes educator (see "Resources") to help you set goals. Even if you plan to use the diet and exercise advice in this book, you should keep in touch with health professionals who can help you monitor your progress.

Q: I don't have type 2 diabetes right now; but I have several relatives who do, and I developed gestational diabetes during my last pregnancy. What should I do?

Both gestational diabetes and a family history put you at risk for developing type 2 diabetes later in life. But in some ways you are lucky: You are aware of your risk, and there is a lot you can do. If you are not a regular exerciser, make this your number one priority and get going right away. Studies suggest that the children of people with type 2 diabetes can keep the disease at bay by becoming fit and keeping their body fat at a healthy level. Of course, the other equally important piece is to eat the Good Fat Diet described in this book. If you are healthy and active you may not need a strict calorie limit; following the eating strategies outlined in this book should help you stay that way.

Q: Should women with type 2 diabetes take hormone replacement therapy after menopause?

Like all women, women with type 2 diabetes have to weigh the potential risks and benefits before deciding to take hormone-replacement therapy (HRT). The biggest issues are that HRT increases breast cancer risk and lowers heart disease risk. For many women, particularly women with type 2 diabetes, the risk of heart disease far outweighs the risk of breast cancer. Indeed, new research suggests that women with type 2 diabetes have even more to gain from HRT than everyone else, because they are in greater need of estrogen's protective effect against heart disease. Women who take HRT have better blood sugar control and lower risk of complications. Research also suggests that HRT can be a preventive measure: Women who take estrogen have been found to be five times less likely to develop type 2 diabetes.

Q: If I am at risk for heart disease, but not type 2 diabetes, can I use the information in this book?

Yes, by all means. All of the research on the Mediterranean diet on which the Good Fat Diet is based points to the fact that this eating pattern is ideal for lowering risk for heart disease. If you have high triglycerides and low HDL cholesterol, the Good Fat Diet is preferable to a very low fat diet, which may worsen these two risk factors. However, if your triglycerides and HDL are normal, but you have high levels of LDL cholesterol, a low-fat or very low fat diet, such as the Ornish diet (page 217) may be an alternative.

Q: Whatever happened to the prudent diet?

The so-called prudent diet, which emphasizes the use of margarine and other polyunsaturated fats, is now outdated because it was based on what was known back in the 1960s when it was first recognized that heart disease was becoming a national epidemic. But we have since learned that a diet high in polyunsaturated fats tends to lower the good HDL cholesterol along with the bad; we have also learned that keeping HDL cholesterol as high as possible is powerful protection against heart disease. This is not to say you can never eat polyunsaturated fats—they are widespread in our food supply and they *do* help lower the bad cholesterol—it is to say that the fats you *add* to your food should be monounsaturated.

Q: Why aren't we being told to watch out for cholesterol and why doesn't this book list cholesterol in the nutritional analyses?

If you are careful about the saturated fat in your diet, the amount of cholesterol you eat will also stay low. But keep in mind that what raises the cholesterol in your blood is eating too much saturated fat and too many calories; the cholesterol in food has a relatively small effect. The amount of cholesterol is deliberately not included in the nutritional analyses to get you to focus on what really matters—keeping the saturated fat down and the fiber up. Too many people make the mistake of looking for foods low in cholesterol when many low-cholesterol foods are loaded with the worst kind of blood-cholesterol-raising fats. (Some examples: solid vegetable shortening, stick margarine, many commercial baked goods, and snacks made with hydrogenated oils.) Are these foods cholesterol free? Yes. Are these foods good for you? *No!* Do yourself a favor—stop thinking about the cholesterol in food once and for all. There, that's one less thing to worry about. Now you can focus on what you should eat to lower the cholesterol *in your blood.*

Q: If dietary cholesterol isn't as important as the type of fat you eat, why do some doctors tell their patients to go on low-cholesterol diets?

The term *low-cholesterol diet* should be abandoned, because it is a source of great confusion. Again, cholesterol *in the diet* is not the issue; it is saturated fat, which is by far the most potent raiser of cholesterol *in the blood.* Because the goal of the diet against heart disease is to lower blood cholesterol, it could be called a cholesterol-lowering diet. Better yet, call it the Good Fat Diet because this is how you have to eat to keep the bad cholesterol down and the good cholesterol up, which is what we're really after.

Q: Is the Good Fat Diet a high-fat diet?

No, the Good Fat Diet derives about 30 percent of calories from fat, which is at the upper limit most often used on healthy diets. But the terms *high-fat diet* and *low-fat diet* are relative. To put this in perspective, the average American currently eats about 34 percent of calories from fat, far too much of which is bad fat. Cardiologists often advise their patients to stay well under the 30 percent limit, closer to 20 percent of calories from fat, because limiting all sources of fat helps keep bad fats low too. (And some go all the way to a no-added-fat or 10 percent fat diet, such as the diets of Dr. Dean Ornish; see below.) At the other end of the spectrum, some traditional Mediterranean diets are more than 35 percent fat, with a very large proportion of that fat coming from olive oil, and with most of the other calories coming from legumes, vegetables, fruits, grains, and fish. The most important issue is not how much fat is in the diet, but how many calories are in the diet and how good or how bad that fat is.

Q: Why isn't the Good Fat Diet as high in fat as the Mediterranean diet?

The 30 percent level is more appropriate for the Good Fat Diet—our Americanized version of the Mediterranean diet—because we are controlling calories, and we need room for satisfying amounts of food. This amount of fat allows for a little more lean protein and high-fiber carbs, both of which help people lose weight without feeling hungry. We are also trying to include as many fruits, vegetables, and low-fat dairy products as possible for optimum blood pressure control.

Q: What about the very low fat diets, such as the 10-percent-fat diet of Dr. Dean Ornish?

The research of Ornish has received a lot of attention over recent years; and justifiably so, because he was able to show that his program caused the plaque in the arteries of people with severe heart disease to shrink. But his program has not been shown to reduce the incidence of second heart attacks. Heart patients following the Mediterranean diet in the Lyon Diet

Heart Study (page 42) did have a dramatic reduction in second heart attacks. Researchers suspect that the composition of the diet actually decreased arrhythmias and the blood clots that can precipitate a heart attack.

Some people with heart disease alone may very well benefit from the Ornish approach (if they can stick with the rigid program for life, which is a very big *if*), but people with type 2 diabetes have other concerns. These very low fat diets lower HDL cholesterol, and they have the additional drawback of raising triglycerides, exactly what most people with type 2 diabetes don't need. And because a high proportion of calories come from carbohydrates when fatty foods are kept low, very low fat diets are not necessarily good for blood sugar either. The Good Fat Diet has none of these drawbacks, which makes it the best diet for fighting both type 2 diabetes *and* heart disease.

Q: I have heard that low-fat products are making us fat—now I'm really confused. Are they good or are they bad?

The problem lies with the low-fat treats—the cakes, cookies, frozen desserts, and snack bars—which are usually high in calories, because the fat has been replaced with refined carbohydrates. People gain weight, because they tend to overdo it with treats that are low-fat or fat-free (page 55).

On the other hand, not all reduced-fat products are bad. As a group, reduced-fat dairy products can make a great contribution to a healthy diet, and here lower fat usually does mean lower calories and definitely less saturated fat. Low-fat mayonnaise is another truly useful product; you can cut the calories in a tuna salad sandwich by switching from regular mayo. Besides, you're not likely to see people polishing off a whole jar of low-fat mayonnaise in one sitting, which can easily happen with a pint of low-fat premium ice cream.

The bottom line is to use low-fat products wisely, namely to save calories and lower saturated fat. And keep in mind that processed junk food is no better for you when it's loaded with fat and refined carbs than when it has just refined carbs. When you deserve a treat, why not go for the real thing? How about really good cookies made with quality chocolate, toasted hazelnuts, and whole grains? (See Chapter 18 for some ideas.)

Q: What about salt? How much should I worry about it?

Salt is more or less of a concern, depending on who you are. Some people are sensitive to the amount of sodium in the diet, and some people are not. Unfortunately, other than trial and error, there's no easy way to find out. But if you have hypertension—or if you would like to prevent it—you should probably think about the things that *lower* blood pressure as much as or more than you worry about salt. Number one: Losing weight lowers blood pressure because it lessens the burden of pumping blood over the miles of blood vessels it takes to get to where it's going. Exercise lowers blood pressure whether you lose weight or not, because it helps keep the arteries more open and more flexible.

And remember that the DASH study has shown that a diet rich in fruits, vegetables, and low-fat dairy products lowers blood pressure even when weight and sodium are kept constant. This study supports other findings that foods rich in the minerals potassium, magnesium, and calcium help keep blood pressure down. Whether you need special medications or not, these strategies are all important to help maintain a healthy blood pressure and lower your risk of stroke. Because high blood pressure is such a part of the insulin resistance syndrome, the DASH study has special meaning for people with type 2 diabetes. It means that throwing the salt shaker away is not the way to control your blood pressure (far more sodium comes from processed foods anyway); eating a diet rich in fruits, vegetables, and low-fat dairy products is.

Q: What about artificial sweeteners?

You can assume that any artificial sweetener approved by the Food and Drug Administration (FDA) is likely to be safe in moderate amounts, so using them is a personal choice. However, according to the American Diabetes Association, sugar is okay in moderation and should be counted the same as any other carbohydrates. As long as your overall diet is not too high in calories and is rich in nutrients, fiber, and the right amount of good fats, there is no reason to keep real sugar out of your life completely. The recipes in this book use small amounts of sugar to show you how it can be part of a healthy diet. On the other hand, if you want to use artificial sweeteners to shave calories when you can, this is perfectly okay too.

Q: Do I have to drink skim milk every day, or is it okay to save those calories for something else and take calcium supplements?

This is a very good question, and the answer is that you should include milk in your diet if you possibly can because getting nutrients from food is always better than relying on supplements. Foods like nonfat milk and yogurt contain a complicated brew of nutrients and other natural substances that work together to protect and nourish the body. For example, studies have shown that eating dairy products helps keep blood pressure normal; and researchers suspect it is because dairy products contain just the right mix of calcium, vitamins, and other minerals, which may all work together to lower blood pressure.

Q: How much vitamin E should I take, and why can't I just depend on my multiple supplement for extra vitamin E?

Most multiple supplements contain the current recommended amount of vitamin E; and while this is enough to prevent a deficiency, it may not be enough to offer maximal protection against heart disease. The exact amount needed is not known, so even your doctor has to make an educated guess based on what is known. To be honest, taking large doses of vitamin E is really like taking a drug, because the amount is far more than the amount anyone could possibly get from food alone. One would have to drink vegetable oil by the cupful. However, vitamin E may very well turn out to be one of the best drugs around, because it is cheap and effective and, so far, has none of the negative side effects associated with other drugs.

Here are some reference points to help you decide how much to take: The Daily Value is 10 milligrams; the amount found to reduce prostate cancer risk is 50 milligrams; the amount shown to boost the immune system in people over sixty-five is 200 milligrams; the amount used in heart disease studies has been at least 100 milligrams, but usually 400 milligrams. Cardiologists often use 400 milligrams of vitamin E for people at risk for heart disease. The best amount for you is something you and your doctor should decide.

Q: My multiple supplement does not contain chromium, and I understand chromium may be useful for people with type 2 diabetes.

A varied diet should contain enough chromium to meet the body's needs; however, some researchers believe that people with type 2 diabetes have higher requirements than everyone else. Chromium is a trace nutrient that helps maintain insulin sensitivity (page 81), and some research suggests that chromium supplements help lower blood sugar in people with type 2 diabetes. The American Diabetes Association does not recommend chromium supplements, because there are still questions that need to be answered through ongoing research.

Q: I am concerned about reports that a substance called homocysteine can damage arteries, just like cholesterol. Is this true, and should I be taking a folate supplement to lower my homocysteine levels?

Yes, recent research suggests that high homocysteine does appear to be a risk factor for heart disease just like high cholesterol, which may help explain why people with low cholesterol sometimes have heart attacks (page 12). It is also true that the B vitamin folate (folic acid) helps keep homocysteine at safe levels in the blood. Taking a daily multivitamin is an excellent way to make sure you're getting the recommended level of 400 micrograms of folate. This is particularly important, because studies suggest that most people still fall short of this level even with a new government program to fortify grain products with folate. It is better to get your folate from a multiple supplement, because it also contains vitamins B_6 and B_{12}, which assist folate in maintaining safe homocysteine levels.

Q: Soybean oil contains omega-3 fatty acids, so why isn't it listed with the good fats?

True, soybean oil is a source of omega-3 fatty acids, about half the amount in canola oil. But because most of the rest of its fatty acids are polyunsaturated rather than monounsaturated, its ratio of omega-6s to omega-3s is quite high. The other problem is that, at the present time, most of the soybean oil in our food supply is hydrogenated; and wherever you have hydrogenated fats, you also have trans fats, which should be avoided as much as possible.

Q: Isn't the Good Fat Diet more expensive than the typical American diet?

It may seem that way when you're stocking your pantry with new ingredients, such as roasted red peppers in a jar and a gallon of olive oil. But if you're eating a typical American diet now, these foods are really a good deal in comparison. At Boston University researchers planning a large multicenter study, similar to the Lyon Diet Heart Study, compared what people spent to go on a Mediterranean-type diet plan to what they were spending on food before. There was no significant difference. You can save money by stocking up on nonperishable items when you see them on sale, or buying them in bulk at a warehouse-type food outlet. I make a monthly trip to one particular supermarket to stock up on their house brand of canned beans and pasta at less than half the price of that of the nearest market, where I regularly go to shop for great breads and produce.

Q: If it's okay to eat a reasonable amount of fat, why are reduced-fat products used in some of the recipes?

Using low-fat and nonfat products is a great way to lower both calories and saturated fat. The best example of this is dairy products. Whole milk contains 8 grams of fat, 5 grams of which are saturated, and 150 calories per cup. Nonfat (skim) milk contains no fat and just 86 calories. So if a person who drinks three glasses of whole milk switches to nonfat, he or she saves 192 calories and 15 grams of saturated fat a day. And if that same person is on a 1,500 calorie diet, 15 grams of saturated fat is nearly the saturated fat allowance for an entire day.

Q: Why do the menu plans call for so much milk and yogurt? I often hear that adults are better off without milk.

There are at least two very good reasons for including dairy products in the meal plans: fighting hypertension and fighting osteoporosis. Research now strongly suggests that calcium in the diet is very important for maintaining a healthy blood pressure (page 84), and there has never been a question that adequate calcium in the diet (and exercise) is important for maintaining bone strength throughout life. Much of the evidence about calcium and hypertension is from studies on calcium in foods rather than calcium in supplements; but if you have to avoid dairy products because of lactose intolerance or an allergy to milk proteins, supplements are certainly the next best thing.

Q: Can I drink 2% milk instead of nonfat milk?

This brings up one of the misleading things about the way milk is labeled: 2% milk is not really low in fat at 5 grams (3 grams saturated) per cup. The 2% refers to the weight of the fat—2 grams per 100 grams milk—and not the calories as you might think. Because milk is mostly water with a relatively small amount of suspended fat and protein, a weight of 2% fat is actually quite high. For comparison, whole milk is 3.3% fat or nearly 97% fat-free according to its water weight.

Q: When you use nonfat yogurt to make Yogurt Cheese Spread, why is olive oil added? Doesn't this add back fat and calories?

Yes, olive oil does add back some fat and calories, but it is safe fat and it is added for a good reason: taste. Nonfat Yogurt Cheese, which is basically drained nonfat yogurt, has a wonderful creamy consistency but it is rather tart. While it stands in well for sour cream or cream cheese in recipes, it needs a little help to stand on its own. One tablespoon of olive oil per cup of Yogurt Cheese does the trick, making it more mellow, and yet adding only about 12 calories and a little less than 1 gram of good fat per tablespoon. So what you end up with is a Yogurt Cheese that is low fat, rather than nonfat; but the small amount of fat you do get is good fat.

Q: Why is a canola oil spread recommended on the Good Fat Diet, and not a spread made with olive oil?

Two reasons: There is currently no olive oil spread that is free of hydrogenated oils, and canola oil has more omega-3 fatty acids than olive oil. In fact, in the Lyon Diet Heart Study, the researchers attributed omega-3s with part of the protection against second heart attacks in the Mediterranean group. And unlike traditional Mediterranean diets, on which people got their omega-3s from eating lots of greens, fish, and nuts, the people on the Lyon study got the majority of their omega-3s from using a canola oil spread. This means that using olive oil, which is higher in monos, for cooking, and using canola oil, which is higher in omega-3s, for baking and in a spread gives you the best of both worlds. In fact, the combination is very close to what worked so well in the Lyon Diet Heart Study.

Resources

AMERICAN ASSOCIATION OF DIABETES EDUCATORS
For referral to a local diabetes educator.

444 North Michigan Avenue
Suite 1240
Chicago, IL 60611
800-832-6874

AMERICAN ASSOCIATION OF RETIRED PERSONS (AARP)
For vitamin and mineral supplements, over-the-counter drugs, and prescription
drugs by mail order; prices are the same for members and nonmembers.

601 E Street NW
Washington, DC 20049
800-456-2277
Web site: www.aarp.org

AMERICAN COLLEGE OF SPORTS MEDICINE
For information about fitness and exercise.

P.O. Box 1440
Indianapolis, IN 46206-1440
317-637-9200
Fax: 317-634-7817
Web site: www.acsm.org/sportsmed

AMERICAN DIABETES ASSOCIATION
For information about counseling and support groups, free information kits,
testing, referrals, and information about local events.

1660 Duke Street
Alexandria, VA 22314
800-342-DIABETES
800-342-2383
Web site: www.diabetes.org/custom.asp

AMERICAN DIETETIC ASSOCIATION
For food and nutrition information, guidance, and referral to a local registered
dietitian.

216 West Jackson Boulevard
Suite 800
Chicago, IL 60606
800-366-1655
Web site: www.eatright.org

AMERICAN HEART ASSOCIATION
For referral to a local affiliate.

7272 Greenville Avenue
Dallas, TX 75231
800-242-8721
Web site: www.amhrt.org

OLDWAYS PRESERVATION AND EXCHANGE TRUST
For information about the Mediterranean diet and other traditional patterns of
healthy eating.

25 First Street
Cambridge, MA 02141
617-621-3000
Fax: 617-621-1230
e-mail: oldways@tiac.net

OTHER WEB SITES
For free access to medical journal topics through Medline: www.nlm.nih.gov

For updates on omega-3 research: www.teleport.com/~jor

For a listing of the glycemic index of three hundred foods:
www.mendosa.com/gi.htm

Selected References

CHAPTER I

Colditz GA, Willet WC, Rotnizky A, et al. Weight gain as a risk factor for clinical diabetes in women. *Annals of Internal Medicine* 1995;122:481–486.

Ernst N, Harlan WR. Executive summary. Conference highlights, conclusions, and recommendations. *American Journal of Clinical Nutrition* 1991;53:1507S–1511S.

Howard BV, Bogardus C, Ravussin E, et al. Studies of the etiology of obesity in Pima Indians. *American Journal of Clinical Nutrition* 1991;53:1577S–1585S.

Knowler WC, Pettitt DJ, Saad MF, et al. Obesity in the Pima Indians: its magnitude and relationship with diabetes. *American Journal of Clinical Nutrition* 1991;53:1543S–1551S.

Martin BC, Warram JH, Krowlewski AS. Role of glucose and insulin resistance in development of type 2 diabetes mellitus: results of a 25-year follow-up study. *Lancet* 1992;340:925–929.

National Institutes of Health, National Institute of Diabetes and Digestive and Kidney Diseases. *Diabetes in America.* 2nd ed. NIH Publication No. 95-1498. Bethesda, MD: NIH, 1995.

National Institutes of Health, National Institute of Diabetes and Digestive and Kidney Diseases. *Diabetes Statistics.* NIH Publication No. 96-3926. Bethesda, MD: NIH, 1996.

Osei K, Gaillard T, Schuster DP. Pathogenetic mechanisms of impaired glucose tolerance and type II diabetes in African Americans. *Diabetes Care* 1997;20:396–419.

Polonsky KS, Sturis J, Bell GI. Non-insulin dependent diabetes mellitus—a genetically programmed failure of the beta cell to compensate for insulin resistance. *New England Journal of Medicine* 1991;334:777–783.

Sims EAH, Horton ES. Endocrine and metabolic adaptation to obesity and starvation. *American Journal of Clinical Nutrition* 1968; 21:1455–1470.

Sims EAH, Horton ES, Salans LB. Inducible metabolic abnormalities during development of obesity. *Annual Review of Medicine* 1971;23:235–250.

Taylor R. Insulin resistance: circumventing nature's blocks. *Lancet* 1996;348:1045–1046.

Wilder LI. *Little House on the Prairie*. New York: Harper & Row, 1935.

Yki-Jarvinen H. Mody genes and mutation in hepatocyte nuclear factors. *Lancet* 1997;349:516–517.

CHAPTER 2

Alfthan G, Aro A, Geu KF. Plasma homocysteine and cardiovascular disease mortality [Research Letters]. *Lancet* 1997;349:397.

American Diabetes Association. Aspirin therapy in diabetes. *Diabetes Care* 1997;20: 1772–1773.

American Heart Association. *Heart and Stroke Facts*. Dallas, TX: AHA, 1997.

Campos H, Genest JJ, Blijleven E, et al. Low-density lipoprotein particle size and coronary artery disease. *Arteriosclerosis* 1992;12:187–195.

Eastman RC, Keen H. The impact of cardiovascular disease on people with diabetes: the potential for prevention. *Lancet* 1997;350(Suppl I):29–32.

Jeppson J, Hein HO, Suadicani DD. Triglyceride concentration and ischemic heart disease: an eight-year follow-up in the Copenhagen male study. *Circulation* 1998;97:1–9.

McCully K. Homocysteine and vascular disease. *Nature Medicine* 1996;2:386–389.

Meigs JB, D'Agostino RB, Cupples LA, et al. Risk variable clustering in the insulin resistance syndrome: the Framingham Offspring Study. *Diabetes* 1997;46:1594–1600.

Morrison HI, Schaubel D, Desmeules M, et. al. Serum folate and risk of fatal coronary disease. *Journal of the American Medical Association* 1996;275:1893–1896.

Nathan DM, Meigs J, Singer D. The epidemiology of cardiovascular disease in type 2 diabetes mellitus: how sweet it is . . . or is it? *Lancet* 1997;350(Suppl I):4–9.

Nesto RWN. Diabetes and heart disease. Symposium at the American Diabetes Association's 56th Annual Scientific Sessions, San Francisco, 1996.

Nygard O, Nordrehaug JE, Refsum H, et al. Plasma homocysteine levels and mortality in patients with coronary artery disease. *New England Journal of Medicine* 1997;337: 230–236.

Pinkney JH, Stehouwer CDA, Coppack SW, et al. Endothelial dysfunction: cause of the insulin resistance syndrome. *Diabetes* 1997;46:S9–S13.

Pi-Sunyer FX. Medical hazards of obesity. *Annals of Internal Medicine* 1993;119(7 pt 2): 655–660.

Ravelli ACJ, van der Merlen JHP, Michels RPJ, et al. Glucose tolerance in adults after prenatal exposure to famine. *Lancet* 1998;351:173–177.

SELECTED REFERENCES   **227**

Reaven GM. Role on insulin resistance in human disease [Banting Lecture 1988]. *Diabetes* 1988;37:195–607.

Ridker PM, Cushman M, Stampfer M, et al. Inflammation, aspirin, and the risk of cardiovascular disease in apparently healthy men. *New England Journal of Medicine* 1997;336:973–979.

Stampfer MJ, Malinow MR, Willett WC, et al. A prospective study of plasma homocysteine and risk of myocardial infarction in US physicians. *Journal of the American Medical Association* 1992;286:877–881.

Stern MP. Diabetes and cardiovascular disease. The "common soil" hypothesis. *Diabetes* 1995;44:369–374.

Suzuki M, Ikebuchi M, Shinozaki K, et al. Mechanism and clinical implication of insulin resistance syndrome. *Diabetes* 1996;45:S52–S54.

Syvanne M, Taskinen MR. Lipids and lipoproteins as coronary risk factors in non-insulin dependent diabetes mellitus. *Lancet* 1997;350(Suppl I):120–123.

Zimmet PZ, Alberti KGMM. The changing face of macrovascular disease in non-insulin dependent diabetes mellitus: an epidemic in progress. *Lancet* 1997;350(Suppl I):1–4.

CHAPTER 3

Ainsworth BE, Haskell WL, Leon AS, et al. Compendium of physical activities: classification of energy costs of human physical activities. *Medicine and Science in Sports and Exercise* 1995;25:71–80.

American Diabetes Association. Clinical practice recommendations 1997: diabetes mellitus and exercise. *Diabetes Care* 1997;20:51–53.

Blair DN, Kampert JB, Kohl HW, et al. Influences of cardiovascular fitness and other precursors on cardiovascular disease and all-cause mortality in men and women. *Journal of the American Medical Association* 1996;276:205–210.

Dunn AL, Marcus BH, Kampert JB, et al. Reduction in cardiovascular disease risk factors: 6-month results from Project Active. *Preventive Medicine* 1997;26:883–892.

Hagan RD, Upton SJ, Wong L. The effects of aerobic conditioning and/or caloric restriction in overweight men and women. *Medicine and Science in Sports and Exercise* 1986;18:87–94.

Klem MJ, Wing R, Hill J, et al. A descriptive study of individuals successful at long-term maintenance of substantial weight loss. *American Journal of Clinical Nutrition* 1997;66:239–246.

Perseghin G, Price TB, Petersen KF, et al. Increased glucose transport-phosphorlyation and muscle glycogen synthesis after exercise training in insulin resistant subjects. *New England Journal of Medicine* 1996;335:1357–1362.

Pi-Sunyer FX. The fattening of America [Editorial]. *Journal of the American Medical Association* 1994;272:238.

Schuler G, Hambrecht R, Schlierf G, et al. Regular physical exercise and low-fat diet: effects on progression of coronary artery disease. *Circulation* 1992;86:1–11.

Skender ML, Goodrick GK, Del Junce DJ, et al. Comparison of 2-year weight loss trends in behavioral treatments of obesity: diet, exercise and combination interventions. *Journal of the American Dietetic Association* 1996;96:342–349.

Yamanouchi K, Takashi S, Chikada K. Daily walking combined with diet therapy is a useful means for obese NIDDM patients not only to reduce body weight but also improve insulin sensitivity. *Diabetes Care* 1995;18:775–778.

CHAPTER 4

Ainsworth BE, Haskell WL, Leon AS, et al. Compendium of physical activities: classification of energy costs of human physical activities. *Medicine and Science in Sports and Exercise* 1995;25:71–80.

American College of Sports Medicine. *The American College of Sports Medicine Fitness Book.* Champaign, IL: Leisure, 1992.

American Diabetes Association. Clinical practice recommendations 1997: diabetes mellitus and exercise. *Diabetes Care* 1997;20:51–53.

Anderssen SA, Hjermann I, Urdal P, et al. Improved carbohydrate metabolism after physical training and dietary intervention in individuals with the "atherothombogenic syndrome." Oslo Diet and Exercise Study (ODES). A randomized trial. *Journal of Internal Medicine* 1996;240:203–209.

Blair DN, Kampert JB, Kohl HW, et al. Influences of cardiovascular fitness and other precursors on cardiovascular disease and all-cause mortality in men and women. *Journal of the American Medical Association* 1996;276:205–210.

Brown MD, Moore GE, Korythkowski MT, et al. Improvement of insulin sensitivity by short-term exercise training in hypertensive African American women. *Hypertension* 1997;30:1–5.

Dunn AL, Marcus BH, Kampert JB, et al. Reduction in cardiovascular disease risk factors: 6-month results from Project Active. *Preventive Medicine* 1997;26:883–892.

Horton ES. Metabolic aspects of exercise and weight reduction. *Medicine and Science in Sports and Exercise* 1986;18:10–18.

Klem MJ, Wing R, Hill J, et al. A descriptive study of individuals successful at long-term maintenance of substantial weight loss. *American Journal of Clinical Nutrition* 1997;66:239–247.

Pate RR, Pratt M, Blair SN, et al. Physical activity and public health: a recommendation from the Centers of Disease Control and Prevention and the American College of Sports Medicine. *Journal of the American Medical Association* 1995;273:420–427.

Perseghin G, Price TB, Petersen KF, et al. Increased glucose transport-phosphorlyation and muscle glycogen synthesis after exercise training in insulin resistant subjects. *New England Journal of Medicine* 1996;335:1357–1362.

Pi-Sunyer FX. The fattening of America [Editorial]. *Journal of the American Medical Association* 1994;272:238.

Schuler G, Hambrecht R, Schlierf G, et al. Regular physical exercise and low-fat diet: effects on progression of coronary artery disease. *Circulation* 1992;86:1–11.

Skender ML, Goodrick GK, Del Junce DJ, et al. Comparison of 2-year weight loss trends in behavioral treatments of obesity: diet, exercise and combination interventions. *Journal of the American Dietetic Association* 1996;96:342–349.

Yamanouchi K, Takashi S, Chikada K. Daily walking combined with diet therapy is a useful means for obese NIDDM patients not only to reduce body weight but also improve insulin sensitivity. *Diabetes Care* 1995;18:775–778.

CHAPTER 5

Berry E, Eisenberg S, Friedlander Y, et al. Effects of diets rich in monounsaturated fatty acids on plasma lipoproteins—the Jerusalem Nutrition Study II. Monounsaturated fatty acids vs. carbohydrates. *American Journal of Clinical Nutrition* 1992;56:394–403.

DeLorgeril M, Renaud S, Mamelle N. Mediterranean alpha-linolenic acid-rich diet in secondary prevention of coronary heart disease. *Lancet* 1994;343:1454–1459.

Felton CV, Crook DC, Davies MJ, et al. Dietary polyunsaturated fatty acids and composition of human aortic plaques. *Lancet* 1994;344:1195–1196.

Franz MJ, Horton ES, Bantle JP, et al. Nutrition principles for the management of diabetes and related complications. *Diabetes Care* 1994;17:490–518.

Hegsted DM, Ausman LM, Johnson JA, et al. Dietary fat and serum lipids: an evaluation of the experimental data. *American Journal of Clinical Nutrition* 1993;57:875–883.

Hiser E. The Mediterranean diet and cardiovascular disease. *Journal of Cardiopulmonary Rehabilitation* 1995;15:179–182.

Keys A. Coronary heart disease in seven countries. *Circulation* 1970;41(S1):1–211.

Keys A, Menotti A, Karovenen MJ, et al. The diet and the 15-year death rate in the Seven Countries Study. *American Journal of Epidemiology* 1986;124:903–915.

Mattson FH, Grundy SM. Comparison of monounsaturated fatty acids and carbohydrates for lowering plasma cholesterol. *New England Journal of Medicine* 1986;314:745–748.

Pagman A, Bananome A. Position statement: monounsaturated fatty acids in human nutrition. *Journal of the American College of Nutrition* 1992;56:394–403.

Riccardi G, Rivellese A. Diabetes. In: Spiller G, ed. *The Mediterranean Diets in Health and Disease.* New York: Van Nostrand Reinhold, 1991:277–286.

Sacks FM, McManus K. Weight reduction: a comparison of a high unsaturated fat diet with nuts versus a low-fat diet. Abstract presented at the meetings of the Society of Experimental Biology, San Francisco, 1998.

Spiller G. Physiological effects of monounsaturated oils. In: Spiller G, ed. *The Mediterranean Diets in Health and Disease.* New York: Van Nostrand Reinhold, 1991:182–191.

Trichopoulou A, Lagiou P, Trichopoulos D. Traditional Greek diet and coronary heart disease. *Journal of Cardiovascular Risk* 1994;1:9–15.

Ulbricht TLV, Southgate DAT. Coronary heart disease: seven dietary factors. *Lancet* 1991;338:985–992.

Willet W. Diet and health: what should we eat? *Science* 1994;264:532–537.

CHAPTER 6

Andersson H. Effects of carbohydrates on the excretion of bile acids, cholesterol, and fat from the small bowel. *American Journal of Clinical Nutrition* 1994;59(Suppl): 785S–789S.

Jenkins DJA, Leeds AR, Gassull MA, et al. Decrease in post-prandial insulin and glucose concentrations by guar and pectin. *Annals of Internal Medicine* 1977;86:20–23.

Jenkins DJA, Wolever T, Nineham R, et al. Guar crispbread in the diabetic diet. *British Medical Journal* 1978;2:1744–1746.

Kushi LH, Meyer KA, Folson AR. Dietary fat and fiber and death from coronary heart disease in women [Abstract]. *Abstracts of the 38th Annual Conference on Cardiovascular Disease Epidemiology and Prevention,* Santa Fe, 1998;16:3.

Marlett JA. Content and composition of dietary fiber in 117 frequently consumed foods. *Journal of the American Dietetic Association* 1992;92:175–186.

Miller JCB. The importance of glycemic index in diabetes. *American Journal of Clinical Nutrition* 1994;59(Suppl):747S–752S.

Pennington JAT. *Bowes and Church's Food Values of Portions Commonly Used.* New York: Harper & Row, 1987.

Pereira MA, Jacobs DR, Kushi, L, et al. Whole grain consumption, body weight, fat distribution, and insulin in a bi-racial cohort of young adults: the CARDIA Study [Abstract]. *Abstracts of the 38th Annual Conference on Cardiovascular Disease Epidemiology and Prevention,* Santa Fe, 1998;16:3.

Pick ME, Hawrysh ZJ, Gee MI, et al. Oat bran concentrate bread products improve long-term control of diabetes: a pilot study. *Journal of the American Dietetic Association* 1996;96:1254–1261.

Pietinen P, Rimm E, Korhonen P, et al. Intake of dietary fiber and risk of coronary heart disease in a cohort of Finnish men. *Circulation* 1996;94:2720–2727.

Salmeron J, Manson JE, Stampfer MJ, et al. Dietary fiber, glycemic load and risk of non-insulin-dependent diabetes mellitus in women. *New England Journal of Medicine* 1997;277:472–477.

Simpson HCR, Lousley S, Geekie M, et al. A high carbohydrate leguminous fibre diet improves all aspects of diabetic control. *Lancet* 1981;1:1–6.

Trowell HC. Dietary-fiber hypothesis of the etiology of diabetes mellitus. *Diabetes* 1975;24:762–765.

Wolever TMS, Jenkins AL, Sapadafora PJ. Grains, legumes, fruits and vegetables: lente carbohydrate sources in the Mediterranean diet. In: Spiller GA, ed. *The Mediterranean Diets in Health and Disease.* New York: Van Nostrand Reinhold, 1991:160–181.

CHAPTER 7

Bjorck I, Granfeldt Y, Liljeberg H, et al. Food properties affecting the digestion and absorption of carbohydrates. *American Journal of Clinical Nutrition* 1994;59(Suppl):699S–705S.

Connor W, Connor, S, Katan MB, et al. Should a low-fat, high-carbohydrate diet be recommended for everyone? [Clinical Debate]. *New England Journal of Medicine* 1997; 337:562–567.

Coulston AC, Reaven GM. Much ado about (almost) nothing. *Diabetes Care* 1997;20:1–8.

Daly ME, Vale C, Wallace M, et al. Dietary carbohydrates and insulin sensitivity: a review of the evidence and clinical implications. *American Journal of Clinical Nutrition* 1997;66:1072–1085.

Franz MJ, Horton ES, Bantle JP, et al. Nutrition principles for the management of diabetes and related complications. *Diabetes Care* 1994;17:490–518.

Garg A, Bantle J, Henry RR, et al. Effects of varying carbohydrate content of diet in patients with non-insulin dependent diabetes mellitus. *Journal of the American Medical Association* 1994;271:1421–1428.

Holt SHA, Brand Miller JCB, Petocz P. An insulin index of foods: the insulin demand generated by 1000-kJ portions of common foods. *American Journal of Clinical Nutrition* 1997;66:1264–1276.

Jenkins DJA, Jenkins AL, Wolever TMS, et al. Low glycemic index: lente carbohydrates and physiological effects of altered food frequency. *American Journal of Clinical Nutrition* 1994;59(Suppl):706S–709S.

Jenkins DJA, Wolever TMS, Taylor RH, et al. Glycemic index of foods a physiological basis for carbohydrate exchange. *American Journal of Clinical Nutrition* 1981;34:362–366.

Miller JCB. The importance of glycemic index in diabetes. *American Journal of Clinical Nutrition* 1994;59(Suppl):747S–752S.

Pereira MA, Jacobs DR, Kushi L, et al. Whole grain consumption, body weight, fat distribution, and insulin in a bi-racial cohort of young adults: the CARDIA Study [Abstract]. *Abstracts of the 38th Annual Conference on Cardiovascular Disease Epidemiology and Prevention*, Santa Fe, 1998;16:3.

Salmeron J, Manson JE, Stampfer MJ, et al. Dietary fiber, glycemic load and risk of non-insulin-dependent diabetes mellitus in women. *New England Journal of Medicine* 1997;277:472–477.

CHAPTER 8

Christiansen E, Schnider S, Palmvig B, et al. Intake of diet high in trans monounsaturated fatty acids or saturated fatty acids. Effects on postprandial insulinemia and glycemia in obese patient with NIDDM. *Diabetes Care* 1997;20:881–886.

Daviglus, ML, Stamler J, Orencia AJ, et al. Fish consumption and the 30-year risk of myocardial infarction. *New England Journal of Medicine* 1997;336:1046–1053.

DeLorgeril M, Salen P, Martin JL, et al. Effect of a Mediterranean type of diet on the rate of cardiovascular complications in patients with coronary artery disease. Insights into the cardioprotective effect of certain nutriments. *Journal of the American College of Cardiology* 1996;28:1109–1110.

Gogos CA, Ginopoulos O, Salsa B, et al. Dietary omega-3 polyunsaturated fatty acids plus vitamin E restore immunodeficiency and prolong survival for severely ill patients with generalized malignancy: a randomized control trial. *Cancer* 1998;82:395–402.

Holman RT. The slow discovery of the importance of omega-3 essential fatty acids in human health. *Journal of Nutrition* 1998;128:427S–433S.

Kohlmeier L, Simonsen N, Van Veer P, et al. Adipose tissue trans fatty acids and breast cancer in the European Community Multicenter Study on Antioxidants, Myocardial Infarction, and Breast Cancer. *Cancer Epidemiological Biomarkers & Prevention* 1997;6:705–710.

Low CC, Grossman EB, Gumbier B. Potentiation of effects of weight loss by monounsaturated fatty acids in obese NIDDM patients. *Diabetes* 1996;45:569–575.

Mann JI. The role of nutritional modification in the prevention of macrovascular complications of diabetes. *Diabetes* 1997;46:S125–S130.

Parfitt VJ, Desomeaux K, Bolton CH, et al. Effects of high monounsaturated and polyunsaturated fat diets on plasma lipoproteins and lipid peroxidation in type 2 diabetes mellitus. *Diabetes Medicine* 1994;11:85–91.

Simonsen N, van Verr P, Strain JJ, et al. Adipose tissue omega-3 and omega-6 fatty acid content and breast cancer in the EURAMIC study. European Community Multicenter Study on Antioxidants, Myocardial Infarction, and Breast Cancer. *American Journal of Epidemiology* 1998;147:342–352.

Simopoulus AP. Omega-3 fatty acids in health and disease and in growth and development. *American Journal of Clinical Nutrition* 1991;54:438–463.

Simopoulos AP, Robinson JR. *The Omega Plan.* New York: HarperCollins, 1998.

Storlien LH. Skeletal muscle, membrane lipids, and insulin resistance. *Lipids* 1996;31S: 261S–265S.

Storlien LH, Krisketos AD, Calvert GD, et al. Fatty acids, triglycerides and syndromes of insulin resistance. *Prostaglandins, Leukotrienes, Essential Fatty Acids* 1997;57:379–385.

Sundam K, Ismail A, Hayes KC, et al. Trans (elaidic) fatty acids adversely affect the lipoprotein profile relative to specific saturated fatty acids in humans. *Journal of Nutrition* 1997;127:514S–520S.

Walker KZ, O'Dea K, Nicholson GC, et al. Dietary composition, body weight and NIDDM. *Diabetes Care* 1995;18:401–402.

Zock PL, Katan MB. Trans fatty acids, lipoproteins, and coronary risk. *Canadian Journal of Physiology and Pharmacology* 1997;75:211–226.

CHAPTER 9

Adams JS, Lee G. Gains in bone mineral density with resolution of vitamin D intoxication. *Annals of Internal Medicine* 1997;127:203–206.

Anderson RA, Cheng N, Bryden NA, et al. Elevated intakes of supplemental chromium improve glucose and insulin variables in individuals with type 2 diabetes. *Diabetes* 1997;46:1786–1791.

Baker DE, Campbell RK. Vitamin and mineral supplementation in patients with diabetes mellitus. *Diabetes Educator* 1992;18:420–427.

Bendich A, Machlin TK. Safety of oral intake of vitamin E. *American Journal of Clinical Nutrition* 1988;48:612–619.

Blanchard J, Tozer TN, Rowland M. Pharmacokinetic perspectives on megadoses of ascorbic acid. *American Journal of Clinical Nutrition* 1997;66:1165–1171.

Blumberg J. Nutritional needs of seniors. *Journal of the American College of Nutrition* 1997;16:517–523.

Bursel S, Clermont A, Aiello LP, et al. Vitamin E treatment normalizes retinal blood flow and improves renal function in IDDM patients: results of a double masked crossover clinical trial. *Diabetes* 1998;47S:A100.

Chen MS, Hutchinson ML, Pecoraro RE, et al. Hyperglycemia-induced intracellular depletion of ascorbic acid in human mononuclear leukocytes. *Diabetes* 1983;32:1078–1081.

Cox BD, Butterfield WJH. Vitamin C supplements and diabetic cutaneous capillary fragility. *British Medical Journal* 1975;3:205–206.

Cunningham JJ, Mearke PL, Brown RG. Vitamin C and aldose reductase inhibitor that normalizes sorbitol in insulin-dependent diabetes mellitus. *Journal of the American College of Nutrition* 1994;13:344–350.

Davie SJ, Gould BJ, Yudkin JS. Effect of vitamin C on glycosylated proteins. *Diabetes* 1992;41:167–173.

Dawson-Hughes B, Harris SS, Krall EA, et al. Effect of calcium and vitamin D supplementation on bone density in men and women 65 years of age and older. *New England Journal of Medicine* 1997;337:670–676.

Fleming DJ, Jacques PF, Wilson PWF, et al. Heme and supplemental iron intake increases the risk of high iron stores in a free-living elderly population: the Framingham Heart Study. Paper presented at the American Society of Experimental Biology meetings, San Francisco, 1998.

Fuller CJ, Chandalia M, Garg A, et al. RRR-alphatocopherol acetate supplementation at pharmacologic doses decreases low-density-lipoprotein oxidative susceptibility but not protein glycation in patients with diabetes mellitus. *American Journal of Clinical Nutrition* 1996;63:753–759.

Heinonen OF, Albanes D, Virtamo J, et al. Prostate cancer and supplementation with alpha-tocopherol and beta-carotene: incidence and mortality in a controlled trial. *Journal of the National Cancer Institute* 1998;90:440–446.

Jain S, Krueger KS, McVie R, et al. Relationship of blood thromboxane-B2 (TxB2) with lipid peroxides (LP) and effect of vitamin E supplementation on TxB2 and LP levels in type-1 diabetic patients. *Diabetes* 1998;47S:A314–318.

Jennings PE, Chirico S, Jones AF, et al. Vitamin C metabolites and microangiopathy in diabetes mellitus. *Diabetes Research* 1987;6:151–154.

Jialal I, Fuller CJ, Huet BA. The effect of alphatocopherol supplementation on LDL oxidation: A dose-response study. *Arteriosclerosis and Thrombovascular Biology* 1995;15:190–198.

McAlison TE, Felson DT, Zhang Y. Relation of dietary intake of serum levels of vitamin D to progression of osteoarthritis of the knee among participants in the Framingham Study. *Annals of Internal Medicine* 1996;125:353–359.

Morrison HI, Schaubel D, Desmeules M, et al. Serum folate and risk of fatal coronary heart disease. *Journal of the American Medical Association* 1996;275:1893–1896.

National Academy of Sciences National Research Council. *Recommended Dietary Allowances*. 10th ed. Washington, DC: National Academy Press, 1989.

Paolisso G, Balbi V, Volpe C. Metabolic benefits deriving from chronic vitamin C supplementation in aged non-insulin dependent diabetics. *Journal of the American College of Nutrition* 1995;14:387–392.

Paolisso G, D'Amore AD, Giugliano D, et al. Pharmacologic doses of vitamin E improve insulin action in healthy subjects and non-insulin-dependent diabetic patients. *American Journal of Clinical Nutrition* 1993;57:650–656.

Reaven PD, Herold, DA, Barnett J, et al. Effects of vitamin E on susceptibility of low density lipoprotein and low density lipoprotein subfractions to oxidation and on protein glycation in NIDDM. *Diabetes Care* 1995;18:807–816.

Rimm EB, Stampfer JJ, Ascherio A, et al. Vitamin E supplementation and risk of coronary heart disease in men. *New England Journal of Medicine* 1993;328:1450–1455.

Rush D. Periconceptional folate and neural tube defects. *American Journal of Clinical Nutrition* 1994;59(Suppl):511S–516S.

Seddon JM, Ajani UA, Sperduto RD, et al. Dietary carotenoids, vitamins A, C, and E, and advanced age-related macular degeneration. *Journal of the American Medical Association* 1994;272:1413–1420.

Selhub J, Jacques PF, Bostom AG, et al. Association between plasma homocysteine concentrations and extracranial carotid-arterey stenosis. *New England Journal of Medicine* 1995;332:286–291.

Stampfer MJ, Hennekens CH, Manson JE, et al. Vitamin E consumption and risk of coronary disease in women. *New England Journal of Medicine* 1993;328:1450–1456.

Stampfer MJ, Malinow MR, Willet WC, et al. A prospective study of plasma homocysteine and risk of myocardial infarction in US physicians. *Journal of the American Medical Association* 1992;268:877–881.

Yoshida H, Ishikawa T, Nakamura H. Vitamin E/lipid peroxide ratio and susceptibility of LDL to oxidative modification in non-insulin-dependent diabetes mellitus. *Arteriosclerosis and Thrombovascular Biology* 1997; 17:1438–1446.

CHAPTER 10

Anderssen S, Holme I, Urdal P, et al. Diet and exercise intervention have favourable effects on blood pressure in mild hypertensives: the Oslo Diet and Exercise Study (ODES). *Blood Pressure* 1995;4:434–439.

Appel LJ, Moore TJ, Obarzanek E, et al. A clinical trial of the effects of dietary patterns on blood pressure. *New England Journal of Medicine* 1997;336:1117–1124.

Christiansen C, Thomsen C, Ramussen O, et al. Effect of alcohol on glucose, insulin, free fatty acid and triacylglycerol responses to a light meal in non-insulin-dependent diabetic subjects. *British Journal of Nutrition* 1994;71:449–454.

Kiechl S, Willeit J, Poewe W, et al. Insulin sensitivity and regular alcohol consumption: large, prospective, cross sectional population study (Bruneck study). *British Medical Journal* 1996;313:1040–1044.

Lazarus R, Sparrow D, Weiss ST. Alcohol intake and insulin levels: the Normative Aging Study. *American Journal of Epidemiology* 1997;145:909–916.

Mayer EJ, Newman B, Quesenberry CP, et al. Alcohol consumption and insulin concentrations: role of insulin in associations of alcohol intake with high-density lipoprotein cholesterol and triglycerides. *Circulation* 1993;88:2190–2197.

Plotkin F. *Recipes from Paradise: Life and Food on the Italian Riviera.* Boston: Little, Brown, 1997.

Rimm EB, Chan J, Stampfer MJ, et al. Prospective study of cigarette smoking, alcohol use, and the risk of diabetes in men. *British Medical Journal* 1995;310:555–559.

Smith-Warner SA, Spiegelman D, Yaun SS, et al. Alcohol and breast cancer in women. *Journal of the American Medical Association* 1998;279:535–540.

QUESTIONS AND ANSWERS

Anderson RA, Cheng N, Bryden NA, et al. Elevated intakes of supplemental chromium improve glucose and insulin variables in individuals with type 2 diabetes. *Diabetes* 1997;46:1786–1791.

Appel LJ, Moore TJ, Obarzanek E, et al. A clinical trial of the effects of dietary patterns on blood pressure. *New England Journal of Medicine* 1997;336:1117–1124.

Bendich A, Machlin TK. Safety of oral intake of vitamin E. *American Journal of Clinical Nutrition* 1988;48:612–619.

Ferrara A, Karter A, Glei LA, et al. Hormone replacement therapy is associated with better glucose control in a multi-ethnic population with type 2 diabetes: the Northern California Kaiser Permanente Diabetes Registry [Abstract]. *Diabetes* 1998;47S:A152.

Kahn SE, Leonetti DL, Boyko EJ, et al. Estrogen replacement therapy is associated with a reduction in disproportionate proinsulinemia in Japanese-American women [Abstract]. *Diabetes* 1998;47S:A156.

McCully K. Homocysteine and vascular disease. *Nature Medicine* 1996;2:386–389.

Morrison HI, Schaubel D, Desmeules M, et al. Serum folate and risk of fatal coronary disease. *Journal of the American Medical Association* 1996;275:1893–1896.

♥

Index

acorn squash, roasted, 142–143
aerobic exercise, 34, 35
  see also exercise; walking
African-American women, 27, 28
alcohol, 13, 40, 87–89
all-season fruit salad, 204
almond(s), 39, 95, 103
  peach smoothie, 188–189
almost-vegetarian main dishes, 162–173
alpha-linolenic acid, 64
Alzheimer's disease, 72
American Association of Retired Persons (AARP), 77
American College of Sports Medicine, 28
American College of Sports Medicine Fitness Book, 34
American Diabetes Association, 29, 81, 83, 87, 91, 94, 200, 219
American Dietetic Association/National Center for Nutrition, 94, 110
American Heart Association (AHA), 43, 87, 91
amino acids, 12
amputation, 36
Anderson, Richard, 81, 202
angina, 16
animal vs. plant food sources, 18–19, 46
anti-inflammatory agents, 12
antioxidants, 14, 38, 73, 80, 150
  see also specific antioxidants
antipasto, vegetable, 143–144
apples, baked, with crunchy topping, 203

apricots, dried, in breakfast cakes, 187–188
Arborio rice, 158
  in basic risotto, 159
  in zucchini risotto, 159–160
arteries, damage to, 11, 12, 13, 14, 63, 72–73
arthritis, 26, 75
artichoke hearts, artichokes, 96–97
  in big salad variation, 131
  caramelized onions and, 145–146
  and shrimp with lemony pasta, 179–180
arugula:
  in spinach salad variation, 139
  in summer tomato salad, 134
Asian diet, 37–38, 54, 63
asparagus:
  in big salad variation, 131
  roasted, lemony, 142
aspirin, 12, 16
asthma, 66
atherosclerosis, 11, 12, 75
autoimmune diseases, 53, 66
avocados, 70

bacon, Canadian:
  in mess o' greens, 135
  in red beans and rice, 166–167
  in red lentil and rice soup, 171–172
baked apples with crunchy topping, 203
baked stuffed peppers, 165–166
balsamic vinegar, 97
bananas, crunchy baked, 212

chipotle peppers, *see* peppers, chipotle
chivey cheese spread, 198
chocolate hazelnut drops, 208–209
cholesterol, blood, ix, 12, 38, 41, 69, 216–217
   diet and, 13, 37, 49, 50, 51, 59, 63, 216–217
   insulin resistance syndrome and, 15–16
   soluble fiber and, 49, 50, 51
   see also high-density lipoprotein cholesterol;
      low-density lipoprotein cholesterol
cholestyramine, 49
chromium, chromium picolinate, 72, 80–81
   insulin sensitivity and, 81, 220–221
cinnamon, insulin sensitivity and, 202–203
collagen, 75
collards:
   in lentils and bulgur with sausage, 170
   in lentils and bulgur with walnuts, 157–158
   in mess o' greens, 135
colon cancer, 51, 75
company dressing, 132–133
cookies, 207–209
cooking spray, 92
Cooper Institute for Aerobics Research, 22
corn, in Med-Mex casserole, 149
corn oil, 61, 63, 67, 69, 70
cottage cheese, low-fat:
   in chivey cheese spread, 198
   in spinach pie, 152–153
   in vegetable lasagna with a bit of sausage,
      167–168
Coulston, Anne, 57
couscous, 39, 59
Cousineau, Ruth, 144–145, 170
crab cakes, 182
crackers, 100
creamy dressing, 132
crisps:
   Parmesan, 195
   pita, 193
cross-training, 35
crostini, 191
crunchy baked bananas, 212
currant(s):
   in breakfast cakes variation, 188
   pecan drops, 207
cycling, stationary, 35

Daily Value (DV), 78
dairy products, 68, 70, 79, 84, 86, 88, 96, 220, 222
Darwin, Charles, 4
DASH diet, 83–85, 92, 107
   foods in, 84, 96, 219
desserts, 199–212
   sweetening in, 200
diabetes, type 1 (insulin-requiring), 1, 53, 88,
      94, 213–214
diabetes, type 2 (adult-onset):
   as epidemic, 1–2

resources on, 224–225
   risks of, 36
   see also specific topics
diet(s), 83
   of industrialized countries, 2, 41, 54, 60
   monounsaturated-fat vs. low-fat, 40–41
   plant-based, 37–45, 54
   see also specific diets
Dietary Approaches to Stop Hypertension
      (DASH) diet, *see* DASH diet
dip, yogurt-mustard, 191
docosohexanoic acid (DHA), 64
dolomite, 79
drops:
   chocolate hazelnut, 208–209
   peanut butter, 208
   pecan currant, 207
drugs:
   for heart disease, 13, 16
   for high blood glucose, 213

early bird walk routines, 31
easy huevos rancheros, 160–161
Eating Well, 25, 42, 129
Edelman, Robin, 35, 96
eggplant:
   and garlic, roasted, spread, 192
   Parmesan, 150–151
   in roasted vegetables and pasta, 148
eggs, 87
   in frittata, 170–171
   in huevos rancheros, 160–161
egg whites, powdered, 105
energy balance, 17–20
energy nutrients, 18
estrogen, 13, 215
exchange plans, 93–94
exercise, ix, x, 9, 13, 21–24, 27–36, 85
   consistency in, 27, 28, 29, 35
   finding time for, 32–33, 35
   insulin and, 8, 27–29, 34
   starting of, 29–30
   types of, 34, 35
   weight loss and, 21, 22, 23, 24, 26, 27–28,
      34, 85
   see also walking
eyes, 9, 73

fasts, 8
fat-free, low-fat and reduced-fat foods, 40–41,
      55, 59, 218, 222–223
fats, 9, 11, 13, 54, 60–70, 108
   in Asian diet, 37, 63
   good, bad and not-so-great, 70
   in Mediterranean diet, 37, 38, 39, 40–41, 43,
      61, 63, 64, 66–67, 215–216, 217
   ridding kitchen of, 92
   see also specific types of fats

insulin, 1, 7, 8, 9, 19–20, 27, 29, 36, 76, 89,
    202–203
insulin receptors, 7, 9
insulin resistance, 7–9, 40, 54
    alcohol and, 89
    fats and, 65–66, 68
    leptin resistance and, 6–7
    nutrient deficiencies and, 76, 81
    physical activity and, 19, 20, 27–29
    in research, 27, 28, 41, 65–66
insulin resistance syndrome, 15–16
insulin sensitivity, 8–9, 27–28, 34, 65, 202–203
iodine, 79, 100
iron, 77

Jenkins, David, 56

Keys, Ancel, 38, 41
kidney damage, kidneys, 9, 36, 73, 80

lemony roasted asparagus, 142
lentil(s), 39, 56
    and bulgur with sausage, 170
    and bulgur with walnuts, 157–158
    red, and rice soup, 171–172
leptin, 6–7
leptin resistance, insulin resistance and, 6–7
lifestyle, 6, 26, 36, 54
lignans, 100
Liguria, Ligurians, 82
linguine:
    in shrimp and artichokes with lemony pasta,
        179–180
    in turkey tetrazzini, 178
lipoproteins, 11, 13–16
    see also cholesterol, blood; high-density
        lipoprotein cholesterol; low-density
        lipoprotein cholesterol
Little House on the Prairie (Wilder), 3
little meat chili, 169
liver, 13, 49
low-density lipoprotein (LDL) cholesterol,
        13–16, 129, 215
    arterial plaque formation and, 14, 63, 72–73
lupus, 66
lutein, 166
lycopene, 150
Lyon Diet Heart Study, 42, 43, 64, 66, 107,
        217–218, 221, 223

McCully, Kilmer, 12
McMannus, Kathy, 40
macular degeneration, 166
Madeira, pears baked in, 201
magnesium, 76, 84, 108, 219
malnutrition, 2–3, 4
manganese, 79
maple syrup, in basic dressing, 132–133

meat, 87, 93
    in baked stuffed peppers, 165–166
    in beans and greens casserole, 163–164
    in chicken cassoulet, 176
    as condiment, 162–163
    in frittata, 170–171
    in lentils and bulgur with sausage, 170
    in little meat chili, 169
    in mess o' greens, 135
    in red beans and rice, 166–167
    in red lentil and rice soup, 171–172
    in vegetable lasagna with a bit of sausage,
        167–168
    in yellow split pea soup, 172–173
meatless main dishes, 147–161
Mediterranean diet, 37–45, 83
    fats in, 37, 38, 39, 40–41, 43, 61, 63, 64,
        66–67, 215–216, 217
    food pyramid of, 85–87
    foods in, 39–40, 44, 82, 83
    heart-protective properties of, 37, 38–39, 40,
        42, 43, 215–216, 217–218
Mediterranean fish bake, 183
Mediterranean pocket, 194
Mediterranean tuna salad, 184–185
Med-Mex casserole, 149
mesclun, in big salad, 130, 131
mess o' greens, 135
methionine, 12
milk, 86, 220, 222–223
minerals, 39, 79
    see also specific minerals
monounsaturated fats, 13, 37, 38, 39, 40–41,
        43, 67, 69, 83, 103, 223
    not-so-good carbs vs., 59
    polyunsaturated fats vs., 61–64, 216
    see also canola oil; olive oil
mozzarella cheese, part skim:
    in Greek pizza, 154–155
    in vegetable lasagna with a bit of sausage,
        167–168
multiple vitamin-mineral supplements, 73–79,
        110, 220–221
muscles, 19, 27, 28–29, 34
mustard greens, in lentils and bulgur with
        walnuts, 157–158
mustard-yogurt dip, 191

nachos, vegetable, 197–198
National Institutes of Health, 6, 65
Native Americans, 5–6, 41, 66
natural selection, 4
Nesto, Richard, 16
Nurses Health Study, 51, 57
nut oils, 61, 70, 86, 95
nuts, 39, 66, 70, 76, 88, 103
    buying of, 103
    see also specific nuts

oat bran, 49–50
  in peach almond smoothie, 188–189
oat bran cereal, 103
  in breakfast cakes, 187–188
oats, oatmeal, 39, 44, 56, 58, 98, 103
  in breakfast cakes, 187–188
obesity, 3–7, 25, 41, 54, 60
  see also weight, weight loss
"obesity gene," 6–7
oils, dietary, 60–70, 95
  comparison of, 62
  see also specific oils
Oldways Preservation & Exchange Trust, 42,
    85–87
olive oil, 37, 38, 39, 42, 44, 59, 61, 63, 66, 67,
    70, 86, 88, 92, 95–96, 104, 223
olives, black, 96
  in antipasto, 143–144
  in Greek pizza, 154–155
  pizza with caramelized onions and, 155–156
olives, green, 95
  in baked stuffed peppers, 165–166
  in little meat chili, 169
  in roasted eggplant and garlic spread, 192
Omega Diet, The (Simopoulos), 65
omega-3 fatty acids, 39, 43, 61, 64–69, 100,
    101, 131, 221, 223
  insulin resistance and, 65–66
  in Mediterranean diet, 64, 66–67, 86
  sources of, 64, 65, 66, 68, 86
omega-6 fatty acids, 65–67, 70, 221
onions, caramelized, 144–145
  artichoke hearts and, 145–146
  pizza with black olives and, 155–156
onions, green, oven-braised carrots and, 141
Ornish diet, 216, 217–218
osteoporosis, 75, 77, 79, 222
oven-braised carrots and green onions, 141
oxidation of LDL cholesterol, 14, 15, 16, 63,
    72–73, 129

palm oil, 70
pancreas, 7, 53
Parmesan, 86
  in beans and greens casserole, 163–164
  chicken, 179
  crisps, 195
  eggplant, 150–151
  in frittata, 170–171
  in pizza with caramelized onions and black
      olives, 155–156
  in zucchini risotto, 159–160
pasta, 39, 44, 56, 58
  lemony, shrimp and artichokes with, 179–180
  roasted vegetables and, 148
  in turkey tetrazzini, 178
  in vegetable lasagna with a bit of sausage,
      167–168

peach(es):
  in all-season fruit salad, 204
  almond smoothie, 188–189
  and cream, 206
peanuts, peanut butter, 70, 96, 103, 104
  drops, 208
  in peanutty hummus, 189–190
pears baked in Madeira, 201
pecan(s), 95
  in big salad, 130
  currant drops, 207
  in spinach salad, 138–139
peppers:
  baked stuffed, 165–166
  see also bell peppers, green; bell peppers, red;
      red peppers, roasted, in jar
peppers, chipotle, 99–100
  in little meat chili, 169
  in red beans and rice, 166–167
peppers, jalapeño, in shrimp and pepper risotto,
    180–181
periodontal (gum) disease, 12
phyllo dough, 152–153
physical activity, 2, 6, 8, 19, 21–24, 86
phytochemicals, 39, 71, 100, 101, 102, 129,
    131
pie(s):
  spinach, 152–153
  strawberry cheese, 209–210
  vegetable, 151–152
Pima Indians, 5–6, 66
pineapple, in winter slaw, 133
pistachios, 39, 95
pita crisps, 193
pizza:
  with caramelized onions and black olives,
      155–156
  Greek, 154–155
plant vs. animal food sources, 18–19, 46
plaque, arterial, 11, 12, 13, 14, 63, 72–73
Plotkin, Fred, 82
plum tart, 205
plum tomatoes, roasted, 146
  in roasted vegetables and pasta, 148
polyunsaturated fats, 13, 43, 65, 67, 68, 69, 216
  monounsaturated fats vs., 61–64, 216
potassium, 79, 84, 108, 219
potato(es), 56, 58
  sticks, roasted, 137
poultry, 86, 174–179
powdered egg whites, 105
  in peach almond smoothie, 188–189
prehistoric humans, body fat of, 4, 58
prosciutto, 105
  in frittata, 170–171
  in yellow split pea soup, 172–173
prostate cancer, 72, 75, 150
protein, 18, 39, 87, 108

prudent diet, 216
psoriasis, 66
pumpkin walnut cheesecake, 211

Reaven, Gerald, 57
red beans and rice, 166–167
red lentil and rice soup, 171–172
red peppers, roasted, in jar, 105, 166
  in Greek pizza, 154–155
  in Mediterranean pocket, 194
  in roasted red pepper spread, 190–191
  in spinach salad, 138–139
  in vegetable antipasto, 143–144
reduced-calorie dressing, 132
refined and processed foods, 37, 40, 42, 69, 88
rheumatoid arthritis, 66
rice, 37, 39, 54, 58
  and black beans salad, 140–141
  red beans and, 166–167
  and red lentil soup, 171–172
  see also Arborio rice
rice, brown, 58
  in baked stuffed peppers, 165–166
rickets, 3
ricotta cheese:
  in pumpkin walnut cheesecake, 211
  in vegetable lasagna with a bit of sausage,
    167–168
  in vegetable pie, 151–152
risotto, 158, 159
  shrimp and pepper, 180–181
  zucchini, 159–160
rye, 98
rye bread, high fiber content of, 50–51

Sacks, Frank, 40
safflower oil, 67, 70
salad(s), 129–141
  big, 130–131
  black beans and rice, 140–141
  Mediterranean tuna, 184–185
  spinach, 138–139
  summer tomato, 134
  zesty three bean, 139–140
salad dressings:
  basic, 132–133
  company, 132–133
  creamy, 132
  reduced-calorie, 132
  roasted garlic, 132
salmon:
  omega-3 fatty acids in, 67, 68, 174
  simple, 181–182
salsa:
  in easy huevos rancheros, 160–161
  in Med-Mex casserole, 149
  in vegetable nachos, 197–198
salt, sodium, 84, 85, 219

saturated fats, 13, 37, 38, 61, 63, 68, 69, 87,
    216
sausage:
  lentils and bulgur with, 170
  vegetable lasagna with a little bit of, 167–168
savory fats, 58
scurvy, 2–3
sesame seeds, 96, 102
Seven Countries Study, 37–38, 41, 42, 66, 107
shrimp:
  and artichokes with lemony pasta, 170–180
  and pepper risotto, 180–181
Simopoulus, Artemis, 65, 66
slaw, winter, 133
small dense LDLs, 16
small meals and snacks, 186–198
smoking, 12, 129
sole, simple, 184
soluble fiber, 48, 49–51, 103
  blood glucose and, 48–51, 54, 56, 57, 98
sorbitol, 75
soup:
  red lentil and rice, 171–172
  yellow split pea, 172–173
soybean oil, 63, 70, 221
soybeans, 63
spinach:
  in big salad, 130
  fresh vs. frozen, 101
  in lentils and bulgur with sausage, 170
  in lentils and bulgur with walnuts, 157–158
  pie, 152–153
  salad, 138–139
  in vegetable lasagna with a bit of sausage,
    167–168
split pea(s), yellow, soup, 172–173
spreads:
  chivey cheese, 198
  roasted eggplant and garlic, 192
  roasted red pepper, 190–191
  yogurt cheese, 196–197, 223
squash, roasted acorn, 142–143
starches (complex carbohydrates), 39, 49, 56,
    200
Storlien, Leonard, 66
strawberry cheese pie, 209–210
strength training, 34
stretching, 34
stroke, 11, 36, 80
stuffed peppers, baked, 165–166
sugar (simple carbohydrates), 49, 53, 55, 101,
    200
summer tomato salad, 134
sun-dried tomatoes, 105–106
sunflower oil, 67, 70
supplements, 71–81, 220
  see also multiple vitamin-mineral supplements;
    specific supplements